A Self-help Book

ENDOSISTER

MAE BETH, INHC

DEDICATION

I dedicate this book to our daughters, our sisters, our mothers, our grandmothers, and our divine ancestors.

Table of Contents:

A Self-help Book   1

Endosister   1

Mae Beth, INHC   1

Dedication   3

Table of Contents: 4

Chapter 1   10

"Welcoming Health"   10

About the Author   14

"Being Empowered"   15

"Finding the Right Support"   20

"Knowing Gradual Change"   22

"Being an Inspiration"   23

"Accepting Our Authentic Journey"   24

Chapter 2   26

"Integrating Nutrition"   26

"Assessing Our Lives"   27

"Healing Our Whole Being"   29

"Taking Care of Ourselves"   30

"Meeting All Our Essentials"   32

Chapter 3   36

"Healing with Food"   36

"Learning About Dietary Theories"   36

"Avoiding Toxic Ingredients"   41

"Spotting Misleading Labels"   45

"Understanding Organic"   47

"Buying Local"   48

"Knowing Humanity"   50

"Understanding Sugar, Fat and Grains"   51

Chapter 4   59

"Boosting the Immune System"   59

"Flushing the Lymphatic System"   59

"Juicing Fruits and Vegetables"   61

"Boosting Immunity"   67

"Knowing Acid VS Alkaline"   68

"Understanding Bacteria and Fungi"   70

"Identifying Candida Overgrowth"   71

"Controlling Candida"   73

"Running Off Parasites"   74

"Healing Digestion"   77

"Understanding Enzymes"   78

"Consuming Probiotics"   79

"Avoiding Gluten"   80

"Avoiding Constipation"   82

"Knowing Natural Antibiotics"   83

"Detoxing the Body Safely"   85

Chapter 5   87

"Minding our Food"   87

"Deconstructing Food Cravings"   87

"Focusing on Abundance"   90

"Minding Our Food"   92

"Eating Mindfully"   93

"Eating Intuitively"   94

"Grasping Emotional Eating"   96

"Comprehending the Energetics of Food"   97

"Food Journaling for Health"   98

"Connecting to Our Food"   100

Chapter 6   102

"Awakening the mind and the spirit"   102

"Loving Our Mindset"   102

"Knowing the Power of Thoughts"   104

"Affirming What We Want"   105

"Having Gratitude"   107

"Practicing Meditation"   108

"Setting Intentions "   111

"Visualizing Health"   112

"Understanding Autosuggestion"   114

"Connecting Our Emotional Pain with Our Physical Pain"   115

"Loving Our Job"   118

"Creating the Ideal Job"   119

"Remembering How to Play."   120

"Siding with Nature"   122

Chapter 7   124

"Having healthy relationships"   124

"Connecting to Our Higher Selves."   126

"Believing What is True"   127

"Having Emotional Independence"   128

"Living Interdependently"   130

"Holding on to Our Power."   134

"Holding Ourselves Accountable."   137

"Having Healthy Boundaries"   139

"Releasing and Preventing Resentment"   141

"Expressing Our True Feelings"   144

"Accepting What Is"   147

"Coupling and Uncoupling Consciously"   148

"Honoring Our Temple"   150

Chapter 8   152

"Nurturing our Womb"   152

"Learning About Hormones"   152

"Dominating Estrogen Dominance"   155

"Caring For our Reproductive Organs"   157

"Living Within Our Natural Cycle."   160

"Being Curious About the Feminine and the
Masculine"   161

"Having Healthy Intercourse"   163

"Healing Sexual Trauma"   165

CHAPTER 1

"WELCOMING HEALTH"

Dear Endosister,

We might have recently been diagnosed with endometriosis, or we have been walking an uneven path of looking one way, but feeling another for some time. We may have been told, "Well, you look great," when inside, we have had deep pain and a diagnosis that contributes to a feeling of utter doom, exhaustion, and hopelessness. We could have already tried every treatment and practice, we could be on the verge of finding that missing link or puzzle piece, or we are just at the beginning of our endometriosis journey. Here is how it may or may not go for us when we become diagnosed.

When we search the internet, we can become daunted by the words "no cure."

However, we probably won't stop there, our innate nature is always seeking to grow, so we scurry through the internet some more, fixating on the word "treatment" to find a possible solution.

Many of us will follow similar treatment plans that we can find on the leading health websites. After a visit to the doctor, what we hear most likely matches what we read online. We may begin to take medications for pain, some that are highly addictive, mentally, if not physically. We know pain medication is not the answer, we don't want to be on them forever, so we might decide to take shots that stop our reproductive organs to see if we get better. If it is not a success, many of us will find ourselves under the knife, in surgery, cutting away at the tissue or lining left in our pelvic cavities.

Endometriosis is caused by the menstrual cycle going retrograde (backwards). Instead of expelling out our cervix/vagina, it expels out our fallopian tubes! The natural lining inside our uterus that we shed monthly during our menses begins lining the pelvic cavity. Rarely, men and children can get endometriosis, and it can be found in the brain and the lungs. Make sense? Not really. We can make the best sense from what we truly know and feel inside our bodies by keeping an open mind and an open heart. Not everything will be valid for us.

If we have gone through a battlefield, avoided it so far, or don't know where to begin, we might have blessed ourselves with a book that shows a possible path of wellness that is kind or kinder to our bodies, offering everlasting results. What is in this book is practical, attainable, and universal information.

This book will ask a lot of questions for self-awareness. It offers the ability to see the information and take it or leave it. It is easy to read, motivating, and unbiased. Depending on where we are at in our journey, we can adjust the rate at which we take in the information. This book is filled with life-changing ideas and inspirations, including action steps. It is intended to help us grow, not overnight, but at a healthy, honorable, pace that works for us.

If we are expecting a quick fix or a laid out nutrition plan, this might not be the right book for us, but if we desire to become open to an integrative health approach, we must be ready to nurture the entire body, mind, and spirit, by addressing all areas of life. This book offers tools that we can access to create a lifestyle and perspective that aligns with our best selves.

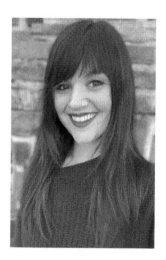

ABOUT THE AUTHOR

Mae Beth is a certified women's integrative nutrition specialist, a writer, a mother, a homeschooler, a hobby farmer, and a farm to table chef. She specializes in women's health education related to women's integrative health, self-help, personal development, nutrition, immunity, auto-immune disease, farm to table cooking, and relationships. After being diagnosed with endometriosis, adenomyosis, fibromyalgia, candida, and leaky gut, Mae Beth now lives her life healthy and well. Her passion is to offer wisdom to other women, using her skills, education, and experiences she acquired along her healing process. Being the person Mae wishes she had during her healing journey, Mae Beth is someone who understands and believes in a positive outcome. If she can inspire or re-inspire us with her gifts of wisdom, Mae is living her purpose.

❖

"Being Empowered"

"I decided to take charge of my health when I realized that the person most in charge of my health was me. I began educating myself on health and wellness and making small gradual changes."
~Mae Beth

We are POWERFUL. Our mind, our body and our soul have infinite power to create change within ourselves, our health, and the world. Sometimes there's a belief inside of us that tells us, feeling better is an unreachable goal. Discovering that there are no known cures for endometriosis can lead to feelings of hopelessness. To go from hopeless to hopeful, we want to believe that achieving better health is something we can reach. We can learn how to take back our power and ignite our energy from within because we are POWERFUL.

As we embrace this reality, we come from such a beautiful feeling of 'Being Empowered.' As we grow stronger, we will see that our journey has many ups and downs. We might even stumble upon negative emotions, including blame and victimhood. Discovering these potential blocks can often make us feel immobile, confused, and in disbelief. In these times, it is inevitable to face non-empowering feelings. However, learning to recognize these feelings, can often ignite incredible change in our lives through recognition. Once we know the difference, we can take accountability and start embracing actions that are known to bring forth, 'Being Empowered.'

During our journey, we sometimes look for the answers in everything but ourselves. Looking outside of us is ok, but we must remember not to forget ourselves in the process. We want to be open and align with our answers that will come together and accumulate from our own authentic body, life, and experiences. Let's take the information that resonates and leave what does not. We can continue to educate ourselves, stay inspired, and experiment. We do not need to hold on to what does not align with our greater knowing. We are empowered. We grow from our own pace and place, not anyone else's.

Transformation might not come overnight, but we do have the ability to make many small changes over time. Growth is growth. Let's be courageous while being easy on ourselves. We can feel like we know it all, and then find that we know nothing. Neither is true. It's a mysterious and individual process where we must keep growing and keep loving ourselves through life's rollercoasters. It does get better if we continue discovering who we are and how we thrive from a compassionate mindset.

Action:

Take a moment to review the Empowered vs. Not Empowered list. Being 100% honest with ourselves, we can create a personal record of areas in our lives where we feel more empowered or less empowered.

In the areas we feel do not feel empowered, let's write down three action steps that we can take in each area so we can feel more empowered.

Empowered

- Open to changes
- Proactive
- Self-accountable
- Self-directed
- Expresses feelings
- Learns from mistakes
- Confronts
- Lives in present
- Realistic
- Sees options
- Develops commitments
- Self-loving
- Values others
- Attends to needs of others
- Balanced lifestyle

Not Empowered

- Not open to changes
- Reactive
- Blames others
- Directed by others
- Fails to recognize feelings
- Defeated by mistakes
- Avoids
- Lives in the past or future
- Unrealistic
- Tunnel vision
- Keeps obligations
- Dislikes self
- Judges others
- Selfish
- Self-centered
- Restricts lives of others
- Unbalanced lifestyle

Being empowered gives us the ability to have more control over our lives. It provides the opportunity to thrive and grow personally. If we are not empowered, we feel helpless, shutout, and unable to move in the right direction. We become powerless.

The following table lists how we can empower or not empower ourselves:

Empowered

- Setting intentions, visualizing how we will act on those intentions
- Keep going with open eyes and being free to change
- Acquiring self-education and skills, so we make changes ourselves
- Noticing when our feelings are true or false, acting accordingly
- Focusing on realistic goals, making small changes

Not Empowered

- Automatically deciding we can't achieve something, feeling defeated
- Having a closed mind, stubborn to change
- Having to rely on others to do things for us
- Believing we can't change our situation ourselves
- Trying to change or do too much at once and being unfocused

Are we feeling our power yet? Sometimes education and information can seem a bit overwhelming, but remember, this is all on our terms. We do what we want with knowledge, and we can find the authentic ways that can help us along our journey. Let's keep an open mind and stay positive!

❖

"Finding the Right Support"

We are loved.
We are safe.
We are worthy.

We develop many fabulous, meaningful relationships in our lifetimes. We are close to our loved ones, and we share our lives together. We hope that when we become weak, we can be lifted by those whom we spend most of our time. We pray for compassion and understanding from those closest to our hearts. However, we find that weakness in the mind and body can test even our most profound relationships. We may find harmony, but if we don't, we must redirect our focus to loving ourselves.

Not everyone will be able to be with our pain, witness our growth, and understand our change. Part of this journey is learning to be okay with this outcome. Try to avoid pressuring those closest to us to resonate with us, or avoid giving them unwanted advice because there are some things in life that our loved ones might not be able to validate or be able to ever understand. Change, whether good or bad, doesn't only affect us personally; it takes time for our closest ones to adjust. It may feel unloving or promote feelings of victimhood if someone isn't as supportive as we want them to be, but we must remember that we are loved regardless, and so are they. We can allow patience, space, and time for growth and change in ourselves and others, while avoiding becoming a victim to a circumstance or a person. If we truly are a victim of an abusive relationship, find the strength to reach out to safety. We are so worthy of it.

It can be helpful to direct loved ones on how to support us by communicating our needs. Often, we need a simple touch, a good ear, a hug, or a conversation about something light, versus serious advice, worry, or pressure to heal. We must speak about our needs through communication to set proper boundaries that encourage us to grow. We all want to feel loved and accepted when we feel inadequate.

Beyond family and friends, it is extremely beneficial to have people in our lives that can relate. We are not alone, and we can learn a lot from each other. This is an abundant time where we are blessed with incredible tools for connection, giving us many opportunities to talk to people with similar circumstances, that have been unavailable in the past.

Online forums, groups, and social media are right at our fingertips. We benefit most by connecting with others that are on healing journeys, to see that we are not alone. We want to learn to relate to those full of healthy inspiration and growth, rather than those who are feeling victimized by their experience. There are millions of people suffering from disease; we can find those who are willing to fight for change and do what it takes to live a quality life. We want to be motivated by those who have healthful insights.

❖

"Knowing Gradual Change"

It is difficult to be patient with our bodies when we are in such pain. We find ourselves becoming fixated on fad diets and health regimens that leave us feeling disconnected, deprived, and less worthy. When we see that it does't work for us, it can cause a lot of emotional ups and downs and keep us from achieving long term health results. We all want fast, we all want now, but an accumulation of small changes in our health is possibly the only way we can create long term results. With gradual changes, we can begin to slowly feel our symptoms lessen as our lifestyle and behaviors change. Slow and steady wins the race.

We can begin achieving small measurable goals by creating simple steps to accomplish them. Creating these steps is a natural process that can be guided and performed on our empowered terms.

As we educate ourselves, lets make this process rewarding and fun. By making positive, healthy choices, we start becoming an inspiration to others that surround us, which might offer feelings of success and gratitude at an early point in our wellness journey. At this point, we could say to ourselves, "Congratulations!" Deciding to take health steps to feel better might be one of the best decisions we can make in our lives because of what we can learn, become, and inspire.

Remember, success is never instant. Every day we get a little bit better, and it eventually all adds up. We are worthy of this knowledge, we are love, we are light, and we believe in us.

❖

"Being an Inspiration"

Throughout our journey, we may start to notice the attention we get from others. If we choose to share our progress, we will more than likely influence many others to make positive changes in their health as well. The inspiration from sharing our process can create a ripple effect and may be very powerful. When we realize what being a role model can create for the people around us and ourselves, our path can feel rewarding.

We want to invite you to be the change and help us inspire the world. As we heal and support each other, we can continue to feel the joy it brings.

Remember, once we become empowered, we can empower others just by being ourselves. Through small changes and the sharing of our knowledge, we will rise above together.

Think about how we can bring gratitude to our situation. What will we do with the knowledge we learn in life?

❖

"Accepting Our Authentic Journey"

Bio-individuality is a term created by Joshua Rosenthal, founder of The Institute of Integrated Nutrition.

Bio-individuality means that there is no one size fits all diet. Meaning one person's diet can easily be another's poison. This theory also implies that what works for someone else might not work for another. We can learn the tools to connect and listen to our own bodies so we can find exactly what will work for us and what won't work for us. We can work on discovering our individual's core needs, identifying what is no longer serving us and remembering that this is our journey and our path. Let's hold on to that power because we are worthy of it.

We are all so unique and different. It seems very limiting to think that we could all adopt a one size fits all perspective.

We all have a different heritage, ancestors, DNA, backgrounds, experiences, minds, bodies, and souls. Every little thing we do in life affects us uniquely and differently. It sure would make it a lot easier to have a one for all manual to our bodies, but it seems that most of our unique nature will remain personal and mysterious.

We can't help but shine with creation just by being us. Our footprint on this earth has a unique individual purpose and naturally offers love to the planet, so we must learn how to be authentic and find our own particular medicine, amongst other creations.

Action:

How do we feel when it comes to our health? Are we feeling empowered? Are there any action steps we can do to empower ourselves more?

How is our level of support? Write down three actions we can take to receive better support from family and external resources. Never be afraid to reach out and speak up; we are not alone. Having a dedicated journal will be very beneficial to have for reflection, notes, and achievements.

"Nobody can go back and start a new beginning, but anyone can start today and make a new ending."
~ *Maria Robinson*

CHAPTER 2

"INTEGRATING NUTRITION"

Integrative nutrition is far more than a diet. It integrates all areas of life and honors them in the same way we accept healthy food in nutrition. These areas of our lives play an essential role in our health and wellness. A meaningful spiritual practice, a career we love, a life with healthy relationships, and enjoyable regular physical activity alongside a healing diet can allow our whole being to flourish.

We find that our day to day lives are affected by our wellbeing, but rarely do we connect our everyday lifestyles to our pain. This concept may be hard for some of us to grasp as our condition can sometimes leave us feeling overwhelmed or stuck. However, this practice can actually free ourselves if approached with ease and an open mind. We would never want anything to get in the way of our growth, especially unintentionally. So luckily, we can use a well known practice to assess our lives and find what areas in our lives need love and attention first.

Here is an activity that can help us to discover ourselves on a deeper level, contributing to a substantial development in personal growth and self-awareness. Enjoy!

"Assessing Our Lives"

Action:

LIFESTYLE ASSESSMENT TEST

Number a sheet of paper from 1-14   1-10 Scale

1. Relationships 3
2. Career/Career environment 5
3. Physical activity 7
4. Nutrition/diet 5
5. Spirituality 6
6. Self-esteem/self-love 4
7. Social-life 3
8. Creativity 8

9. Health 5
10. Home environment 8
11. Education 10
12. Finances 6
13. Mindset 7
14. Play 10

(feel free to add any areas of your own)

Place a number between 1-10 next to each subject, 1 being the weakest and 10 being the strongest area. Remember to grade based on the health of the area rather than status. For example, if we are not married, it does not mean we are weak in relationships; however, if we are in an unhealthy marriage then we will want to grade ourselves accordingly.

After completing the activity, let's take a look at our weakest points. If our relationships are a 3 or 4 and our diet is a 7, we can see how focusing on diet alone might not get us too far. We can take our time and discover what areas in our lives could use some attention. Remember, a weak area can easily affect other areas of our lives. Never hesitate to come back to this activity anytime. A life assessment test is a great tool that will not only mark our progress, but its design is made to help us discover ourselves and grow personally.

❖

"Healing Our Whole Being"

As we begin to discover that health is more than diet alone, we begin to make changes necessary to better our lives. It's time to let go of toxic relationships, find activities we love, open our hearts, get the job we deserve, and strengthen our self-worth by making small changes, and by receiving education. Through this, we regain our power to help ourselves. Making positive changes is a true example of empowerment.

So let's remember that a toxic relationship, a toxic environment, little or no physical activity, and zero spirituality can contribute to pain and suffering. Got it? Good.

Check-in:

How does it feel to have a better look at our life?
What areas in our life need the most love and attention?
Are we feeling anything blocking our ability to grow or change? Where might they stem from, and what could be the reason for limited action or beliefs?
What in our lives is no longer serving us?
Are there activities we can do that serve us to replace what doesn't?
What are our intentions?
Are we feeling empowered?

❖

"Taking Care of Ourselves"

Here are some self-care and lifestyle suggestions beyond diet that we can take into consideration. Remember, these are simply suggestions. We are the ones in charge of our health, and our journey is genuinely authentic. We are the one to decide if there is any benefit to this message. Let's be straightforward with ourselves and begin making changes by directly bringing awareness to them before setting expectations that are too high.

Like we mentioned in "Welcoming Health," we can move mountains by setting small goals and taking little actions while embracing compassion for ourselves. We focus on small changes to keep us from feeling overwhelmed or powerless. If there's something we can't seem to grasp a hold of or don't want to do, it's ok!! We do what we can do and fly with it!

Lifestyle suggestions beyond healthy eating:

- Avoid cooking with microwaves. Use gas when practical.
- Avoid treated water with fluoride and chlorine. Drink and cook with spring water or use a quality filter.
- Learn to chew food for 30 seconds or more for proper digestion and breakdown.

Relationships

- View everything and everyone we meet with gratitude.

- Do our best to stay on good terms with people, especially our boyfriends or girlfriends, husbands or wives, parents, children, brothers, sisters, friends, and co-workers. Communicate with them regularly, either in person or via telephone or email.
  - Who are we not on good terms with? Who would we avoid at a party?
  - Learn to make an enemy a friend.
  - Live happily, focus on what's new and useful.

Hygiene

- Using a hot washcloth to body scrub two times a day can increase circulation. We can also use a skin brush.
- Avoid synthetic clothing and wear 100% cotton when possible, especially undergarments.
- Avoid chemically perfumed cosmetics.
- Use toothpaste without added synthetics and chemicals.
- Avoid excessive jewelry on our body to allow our natural energy to flow and circulate more freely.

Attitude

- Give generously of ourselves and our resources.
- Live each day happily without overly focusing on our problems.
- Sing an uplifting song every day.
- Foster a sense of humor.
- Offer thanks before and after meals.

• Most of all, create a positive attitude, and an enjoyable environment around us, enjoy the process of becoming healthier and happier.

Meditation and Exercise

• Treat ourselves to regular daily quiet time: study, pray, meditate, and recharge.
• Include exercise as a part of our daily life. Experiment with an exercise style that we love, and that works for us.
• Try yoga, Pilates, martial arts, walking, running, bicycling, rollerblading, swimming, dancing, or sports.

Home Practices

• Keep our living space in good order, including the kitchen, bathrooms, bedrooms, and living rooms. We are our home.
• If possible, include large green plants in every room of our homes to freshen and promote the oxygen content of the air.
• Minimize television watching, or at least keep a reasonable distance away from the television.

"Meeting All Our Essentials"

Sometimes we can get so distracted with life that we can easily forget about our essentials. What good is a healthy diet if we fail to get the proper amount of hydration? Essentials include water, oxygen (clean air), sunlight, sleep, and nutrition.

Water

- Composes 75% of our brain
- Regulates our body temperature
- Makes up 83% of our blood
- Helps carry oxygen and nutrients directly to our cells
- Helps convert food into energy
- Removes waste
- Composes 22% of our bones
- Protects and cushions our vital organs
- Helps our body absorb nutrients
- Cushions our joints
- Makes up 75% of our muscles

Clean Air/Oxygen

- Heightens concentration, alertness, and memory
- It gives us energy! 90% of our life energy comes from oxygen and only 10% of what we consume.
- Gives life to the immune system, our memory, thinking, and sight
- Promotes healing and counters aging
- Strengthens our heart, reducing the risk of heart attacks
- Calms our mind and stabilizes our nervous system
- Promotes quicker recovery time
- Crucial for proper digestion and cell metabolism
- Promotes healthy sleep patterns

Sunlight (Vitamin D)

* Known to reverse cancer
* Kills bacteria, disinfects and heals wounds
* Beneficial for skin disorders such as psoriasis, acne, eczema and fungal infections
* Lowers cholesterol
* Lowers blood pressure
* Cleans the blood and blood vessels
* Increases oxygen content in human blood
* Builds the immune system
* Can cure depression

Sleep

* Promotes memory
* Curbs inflammation
* Helps repair our body
* Strengthens immunity
* Reduces stress
* Helps control body weight issues
* Reduces our chance of diabetes
* Minimizes the occurrence of mood disorders

Proper Nutrition

* Strengthens immune system
* Promotes digestive health
* Enhances responses to treatments
* Can help your energy levels and state of mind
* Helps with weight maintenance

- A healthier heart
- Healthy brain function
- Higher quality of life

Source: http://www.integrativenutrition.com

Action:

We can reflect on our progress. Whether we write it down or spend a few moments bringing awareness to it.

What has changed for the better?
What did we learn?
In what ways do we feel empowered?
How do we feel?
What will more education do for us and those in our lives?
What areas in our lives could use more attention?

We got this! Let's give ourselves a big hug. Life is an incredible journey!

CHAPTER 3

"HEALING WITH FOOD"

"Learning About Dietary Theories"

There are hundreds of dietary theories that have scientific data backing them up. We may come across a few in our lifetime, finding ourselves jumping from theory to theory without realizing that eventually, we will run out of options, leaving us with only a kale and quinoa diet. Then we read an article about negative consequences from consuming kale. Is that how we want this process to go?

No way!!!

We can use theory as an inspiration. We mustn't rule out the research of dietary methods; researching theories help us to gain the knowledge we need to experiment. Here are a few nutritional approaches that are worth exploring. The power is in our hands to study and decide what works for us. We can use the tools provided to help guide us through the process. Soon we'll be eating foods we love based on our body's, desires, and positive education vs. foods that no longer serve us.

THE ENDOMETRIOSIS DIET

The Endometriosis Diet is geared towards balancing the excess estrogen levels and prostaglandins in the body known to be a cause of endometriosis. The diet aims to block the bad prostaglandins and increase the good ones.

This diet consists of healthy oils containing omega-3 fatty acids, whole grains (excluding wheat), beans, brown rice, vegetables, fruits, and oatmeal. Foods recommended to modulate estrogen levels are mustard greens, dark green vegetables, broccoli, and cabbage. Foods avoided are red meats, refined carbohydrates, refined sugars, caffeine, chocolate (sugar), dairy, eggs, fried foods, saturated fats and oils, soy products, convenience foods, additives, preservatives, and alcohol. Further research can help us better understand this diet.

THE INFLAMMATION DIET

We all know that endometriosis causes an abundance of inflammation, resulting in pain and discomfort. Pain is typically a response to inflammation in the body. Dr. Andrew Weil, the author of healthy aging, created The Anti-inflammatory Diet. This diet has been proven to influence inflammation, provide steady energy and ample vitamins, minerals, essential fatty acids, dietary fiber, and protective phytonutrients. The general diet tips are to aim for a variety of foods, include as much fresh food as possible, minimize consumption of processed foods and fast food, and eat an abundance of fruits and vegetables.

Exploring this diet on a deeper level and learning how to stop feeding inflammation can be crucial education that supports a healthy, happy body.

CLEAN EATING

Eating clean isn't necessarily a dietary theory because of its flexibility and history. However, it revolves around maintaining a balanced and personalized diet of fresh, unprocessed food, including fruits, vegetables, grains, some meats and fish, and some dairy. The basic principles are to keep it whole, meaning foods that occur in nature, rather than in a factory. Spending time in the kitchen is another aspect of clean eating, as it signifies that restaurant food is more processed and less nutritious. And lastly, it entails eliminating refined sugar and carbohydrates. Clean eating is an approach that emphasizes quality over quantity. Not all calories are created equal. Eating whole foods ensures that we get adequate amounts of essential nutrients and minerals.

A clean eating mindset can always be something we can revert to if we feel confused about diet. We can find that these simple rules can be life changing. Back to nature is back to life.

THE PALEO DIET

The Paleo Diet, also known as the caveman diet, is a diet high in quality animal protein. It is a bit similar to the Keto and Atkins diet. It is known to help with heart disease, auto-immune disease, diabetes, inflammation, and weight loss. This is not a diet low in animal protein, so it may not work for some, though it's possible it may be the one that can work for us or inspire us.

Paleo consists of fresh lean meats, fish, fruits, vegetables, and healthy fats. It also includes eggs, nuts, and seeds. The diet excludes foods like dairy, grains, refined sugars, potatoes, and salt. Over the last decade, The Paleo Diet has become very popular and is a trend followed by many.

VEGETARIAN OR VEGAN DIET

A vegetarian diet has several health benefits if adequately balanced and is nutrient dense. However, just because a food is meat-free, it does not mean it is healthy. On the other hand, a diet containing meat is not always unhealthy. Here's a list of benefits if the individual follows a nutrient-dense vegan or vegetarian diet of unprocessed foods developed with a healthy lifestyle.

When following a vegan or vegetarian diet, it is recommended to test our vitamin D, cholesterol, and iron levels as these can often become low, creating undesired results. Vegetarian diets, primarily vegan, may need supplementation.

Here are some benefits of a vegan or vegetarian diet that could result:

- Better mood, research reveals that none meat eaters have less depression than those who are meat eaters
- Disease fighting, when done right, this diet is low in total saturated fat, and cholesterol, attributed to a higher intake in fiber, phytonutrients, antioxidants, flavonoids, and carotenoids
- A lean figure, as a result of fewer calories
- Less toxicity, food-borne illnesses, antibiotics, bacteria, parasites are more common in commercial meat, poultry, and seafood when compared to plant foods
- A plant-based diet requires less energy and less farmland.
- Longevity, vegetarians have been found to live longer, healthier lives when compared to meat eaters.

Let's feel free to explore dietary theories further and begin experimenting with foods. We want to avoid feeling bad or discouraged if we can't follow an exact diet. There is so much to learn so much beyond theories. With guidance and support we can create change at a pace that aligns with us, while having compassion and love for ourselves. We are so worthy of it.

Action:

Now that we have gone over a few theories, it's time to take the first action steps!

Let's start by doing some research, and pick one theory that connects with us the most and makes the most sense to us.

Let's pick three rules from the diet and put them into action!

We can try this as an experiment for one week, and if all goes well, keep going!

At the end of each week, let's do a self-check-in to see how we feel, and how we are responding to the small changes we have made.

Did these changes bring any positive changes to our health?

Did we see the benefits of these small changes?

What do we like about these changes, and what do we not like?

Is there anything that didn't work well for us?

Is there anything we can do to make things easier for ourselves?

Are we feeling empowered or not empowered?

❖

"Avoiding Toxic Ingredients"

INGREDIENTS TO AVOID

Artificial Flavors- Artificial flavorings come from chemicals made in a lab and offer absolutely no nutritional value. Every artificial flavoring is known to have detrimental effects on our health. Toxicity and cancer can manifest from constant exposure.

Hydrogenated Oils- When oils are hydrogenated, they lose their natural health benefits. Hydrogenated oils are the closest thing we can get to a toxic sludge running through our bodies. If we see "hydrogenated" anywhere on an ingredient list, we might want to run the other way.

Monosodium Glutamate (MSG)- "MSG" is a slow poison which hides behind dozens of names including, disodium guanylate, disodium inosinate, caseinate, textured protein, hydrolyzed pea protein, and many others. It is known to play a role in the development of several disorders, including migraines, seizures, infections, abnormal growth, certain endocrine disorders, specific types of obesity, and neurodegenerative diseases.

High Fructose Corn Syrup- Companies have switched their labels to say corn sugar instead of HFCS because of the number of people finding out how rough it is for the body. It is known to cause insulin resistance, diabetes, hypertension, increased weight gain and known to be made from GMO corn.

Food Colorings- Food colorings, currently all over the market, are linked to disease and cancer. Blue 1 and 2, usually found in candy, processed foods, and drinks, are linked to cancer in rats. The coloring, Red 3, is used to dye red cherries, sweets, and certain baked goods. It is known to cause thyroid tumors in lab rats. Green 3 is a coloring added mostly to beverages and candy, is linked to bladder cancer. Yellow 6, is used the most, in everything from drinks, baked items, lemon candy, to sausages! It has shown to be linked to tumors of the adrenal gland and kidney.

Aspartame- Results indicate that aspartame is potentially a carcinogen. Made up of three chemicals, aspartame contains, aspartic acid, phenylalanine, and methanol. There are almost 100 different health side effects associated with aspartame consumption. We think that may be enough said.

BHA and BHT- Butylated hydroxy anisole (BHA) and butylated hydroxytoluene (BHT) are used to preserve common household foods. Most processed foods that claim to have a long shelf life are often filled with BHA. It is mostly found in cereals, gum, chips, and vegetable oils. They are oxidants, which form potentially cancer-causing reactive compounds in the body.

Sodium Chloride- Sodium chloride, also known as salt, is very far from real salt. Believe it or not, it has almost nothing in common with traditional rock or sea salt. If a food label lists salt, or sodium chloride as an ingredient, we may want to avoid these foods.

Potassium Sorbate- Toxicology reports show potassium sorbate as a carcinogen, showing positive results for mutation found in the cells of mammals. There have been studies that show toxic effects in the organs of animals. Not only should we avoid this ingredient, but we should also eliminate it from our foods.

Soy Lecithin- Soybean lecithin is leftover waste after crude soy oil goes through a cleaning process. The leftover product contains solvents and pesticides. The toxic hexane extraction process is what is commonly used in soybean oil manufacture today. Another big problem associated with soy lecithin is that it comes from the origin of the soy itself. This emulsifier is typically found in ice creams, chocolate, and many processed cream-based products.

Polysorbate 80- Polysorbate 80 has been found to affect the immune system negatively and cause severe anaphylactic shock and can kill life. Toxicology reports have shown that Polysorbate 80 can cause infertility. It can cause changes to the vagina and womb lining, hormonal changes, ovary deformities, and degenerative follicles. A definite no-no.

Canola Oil- Canola, also like rapeseed oil, is toxic to living things, and it can even repel insects. It is highly industrial and not even close to food. The plant is genetically modified with intensive breeding and genetic engineering techniques. It is known to be a significant contributor to inflammation due to an adverse reaction in the body. It's in most processed foods and salad dressings.

Sucralose/Splenda- Splenda/sucralose is chlorinated sugar, a chlorocarbon. Common chlorocarbons include carbon tetrachloride, trichloroethylene, and methylene chloride. Sucralose is a ubiquitous additive in protein mixes and drinks, so beware to all of us who love to add these into our smoothies.

Refined Sugar- Refined sugar changes metabolism, raises blood pressure, critically alters the signaling of hormones, and causes significant damage to the liver. If it's not a natural sugar, we probably shouldn't eat it.

Enriched Wheat/Grains- Enriched grains have undergone a process that zaps out all the nutrients. It's just refined flour that has had a few nutrients re-added to it, but not enough to make any food made from this nutritionally worthy.

❖

"Spotting Misleading Labels"

Food labels can often trigger us to buy foods that may look healthy on the outside, but when we read the ingredients, it can be far from the truth. Sometimes, the label can claim to be free of an ingredient, yet it is replaced with another harmful ingredient. Many labels claim foods to be sugar-free, all-natural, zero trans fats, light, fat-free; however, they may still be damaging to our health.

Labels can seem overwhelming to some, but after a while, we will know our go-to foods, and we will get to know what brands we trust, making the process much more comfortable. Remember, we want to go at our own pace, making small gradual changes. This is a lot of new information and can take some time to put into practice. Let's be easy on ourselves, not expect to be perfect, and do what we can do. It is all on our terms.

Action:

All the information and education in the world will never do any good if we don't act. It's time to get out there and read labels!

Is it time for a bit of a kitchen makeover? What do we have lingering in our fridge that does not serve us for the better?

Start by finding five products that we would typically purchase that are no longer serving our health and wellbeing by reading the ingredients on labels.

Time to find alternatives! Begin by comparing labels at the store and choosing products that have the best interest in our health and wellness.

As we get comfortable with these products and discover healthy products that we love, we can continue to slowly make the changes we are worthy of making. Remember, nobody does this effectively with long term results by jumping the gun. Enjoy the process and enjoy food!

❖

"Understanding Organic"

Consuming organic food reduces the number of chemical pesticides not only in the body, but it also reduces pesticides in the air we breathe, the soil where our food is grown, and in our drinking water. Insecticides are highly linked to auto-immune disease, cancer, asthma, hormone disruption, reproductive problems, allergies, and have far more effects that are harmful to human health. Beyond social effects, pesticides affect animals, our natural earth biology, killing off essential insects, and beneficial bacteria. The earth is our home, and it is our responsibility to keep it sustainable.

Most people can't afford to buy all organic produce, but here is a list of the most contaminated fruits and vegetables that contain the most pesticides and a list that contains the least contamination.

THE DIRTY 14

1. Apples
2. Celery
3. Cherry tomatoes
4. Cucumbers
5. Grapes
6. Hot peppers
7. Imported nectarines
8. Peaches
9. Potatoes
10. Spinach

11. Strawberries
12. Sweet bell peppers
13. Kale/Collard greens
14. Summer squash

THE CLEAN 15

1. Asparagus
2. Avocados
3. Cabbage
4. Cantaloupe
5. Sweet corn
6. Eggplant
7. Grapefruit
8. Kiwi
9. Mangos
10. Mushrooms
11. Onions
12. Papaya
13. Pineapples
14. Sweet peas (frozen)
15. Sweet potato

"Buying Local"

When we buy local, we consume fresher, more nutritious food. Small scale farms take pride in their produce creating higher quality and more variety. Often, crops are shipped overseas just to be packaged due to lower labor costs. Buying local helps out the environment and carbon footprint by using fewer emissions, less packaging materials, and refrigeration. Not only is it better for the environment, but it also creates more jobs and taxes for local communities. A local farmers market is the best place to buy the freshest local produce directly from the farmer himself.

GMO AWARENESS

Genetically modified organisms, also known as GMOs, are plants or animals modified with the DNA from bacteria, viruses or other plants and animals. They are engineering our food to resist highly toxic chemicals that will kill weeds but not the plant itself. GMOs are banned in most countries, yet we are still fighting the GMO battle in America because we are the ones who created them. We suggest further research to obtain a good understanding of GMOs, if we don't already. GMOs are linked to organ damage, immune system disorders, gastrointestinal disorders, and infertility. They also harm the environment, cross-contaminate non-GMO crops, and increase herbicide.

PRODUCE CODES

Have we ever seen that sticker they put on fruit? Ever notice the numbers? These numbers are a code that tells us whether it is conventionally grown, organic, or genetically modified.

A 4-digit code that starts with a 3 or 4 means that it is conventionally grown.

A 5-digit code that starts with a with 9 is going to be organic.

A 5-digit code that starts with an 8 is genetically modified.

"Knowing Humanity"

ANIMAL PROTEIN GUIDELINES

Not all animal protein is the same.

We don't have to live life as a vegan or vegetarian to be aware of factory farming and know what it means. Animals raised in a factory are unhealthy, inhumanely raised, and frequently given hormones and antibiotics. Carnivores might choose to not educate themselves on factory farming, but we don't have to quit eating meat when we acquire this knowledge. One small step would be to start consuming meat that is better quality and much better for our health, the animals, and the planet. It is entirely up to us whether or not we educate ourselves on this not so light subject, but here's a list of guidelines to take into consideration when purchasing or consuming animal protein.

Buy

- Organic grass-fed beef
- Free-range pastured chickens and eggs
- Wild-caught seafood

- Organic grass-fed dairy

Avoid

- Conventionally raised beef
- Conventionally raised chickens and eggs
- Farmed seafood
- Sweetened or processed dairy sources

Check-in:

Feeling educated yet? Overwhelmed maybe? Sometimes information like this can be a lot to take in. It is a lot of information. Who wants to read labels? Let's shine some positivity here for a moment. Remember, simplicity is bliss! We may be thinking, how is this simple? Well, it's as simple as we make it. We don't have to worry about much if we go back to the basics. We can eat whole single ingredient foods and buy organic when possible. This earth is filled with an abundance of fruits and vegetables with many varieties that are endless.

"Understanding Sugar, Fat and Grains"

Sugar, fat, and grains are not all created equal. Refined sugar and sugar substitutes can't compare to natural sugar, processed fats, and animal fats don't compare to natural plant-based fats, and enriched processed grains will never compare to whole grains.

SUGAR

Sugar is one of the leading contributors to obesity, cancer, and disease. Because of its dopamine effects, it is highly addictive.

Sugar can be havoc on a weakened immune system and can feed any type of infection (bacterial and fungal), which can in turn, create uncontrollable cravings. Today, sugar has made its way into almost everything, so we must understand the difference between the good and the bad. However, if we have an infection of any kind or we are battling candida, we recommend temporarily excluding all sugar from our diet, in addition to reaching out to a professional doctor or naturopath.

Whole foods such as fruits, vegetables, beans, nuts, and whole grains contain natural, simple sugars. Sugar from whole foods comes with vitamins, minerals, proteins, phytochemicals, and fiber. Fiber makes a profound difference because it slows down the absorption and its impact on blood sugar. Natural sugars found in whole foods are known as 'good' sugar. When sugar is added to foods during processing, we consume calories without any nutrients or fiber. Sugar that is added sugar is typically unhealthy.

Good Sugar

• Fruit

- Raw local honey
- Real maple syrup
- Coconut sugar
- Blackstrap molasses
- Stevia

Bad Sugar

- Refined sugar
- Added sugar
- Cane sugar
- High fructose corn syrup
- Corn syrup
- Agave syrup
- Splenda
- Aspartame
- Sucralose

FATS

There has always been a debate on whether or not we should be consuming high or low-fat diets. Some of us believe fats play a crucial role. Our bodies are naturally fatty; our liver and organs are oily, and so is our skin. Our bodies may need these fats for proper lymphatic drainage and as a lubricant for our bodies. A diet too low in fats may affect hormones, cause inflammation, and contribute to dry aging skin and hair. Some people believe a low-fat diet works best for their body. It is in our power to find what works for us and makes sense to us.

It's important to know the difference between fats because they are not all created equal. Monounsaturated fats and polyunsaturated fats are known to be good for your heart, cholesterol, and overall health. Trans fats and saturated fats are bad fats, known to increase the risk of disease and cholesterol. Here's a list of good and bad fats that we put together after lots of research, collaboration, and experimentation.

Good Fats

- Olive Oil (cold)
- Grapeseed oil (high heat)
- Coconut oil (medium heat)
- Avocado oil (cold)
- Nut oils
- Fish oil
- Flaxseed oil Foods
- Nuts and seeds
- Avocados
- Wild fish
- Olives
- Ghee
- Animal fats from grass-fed cage-free animals
- Grass-fed butter

Bad Fats

- Processed unnatural fat
- Partially hydrogenated
- Vegetable shortening

- Trans fats
- Margarine oil
- Canola oil (corn oil)
- Rapeseed oil
- Cottonseed oil
- Soybean oil
- Safflower oil
- Peanut oil

OMEGA-3 FATTY ACIDS

For those of you who don't know, omega-3 fatty acids are in good fats known as EPA and DHA. These acids have profound health benefits and are crucial to maintaining proper brain function and inflammatory responses.

Ever feel scatterbrained and unable to focus? Suffer from ADD or ADHD? How about depression or inflammation? We may suffer from an imbalance of omega. It is common for individuals to have an overload of omega-6 fatty acids creating a high omega-6 to omega-3 ratio. A diet high in omega-6 and low in omega-3 can cause many chronic diseases, including autoimmune disease. Omega- 3 fatty acids tend to have potent anti-inflammatory effects, whereas omega-6 fatty acids tend to be pro-inflammatory. Remember, both omegas are essentials; it's the imbalance that causes problems. The goal is to achieve a ratio of 2:1 or 3:1 rather than the average consumption of 10:1 to 20:1 when it comes to an omega-3 to omega-6 ratio.

Some foods high in omega-3 include algae, fish oil or seafood, flaxseed oil or flaxseeds, chia seeds, walnut oil, or walnuts. Examples of foods high in omega-6 are vegetable oils such as soybean, corn, safflower, canola, margarine, chicken, pork, dairy, eggs, and processed foods. Not all fatty acids are created equal, so it is in our power to research more on this subject.

Supplementation is highly recommended for those who may not be receiving enough omega-3 through diet alone. We have seen, heard, and experienced profound benefits from supplementing. Our favorite source is from blue-green algae containing DHA because it is plant-based, and it doesn't promote overfishing our waters. However, high-quality fish oil is another natural supplement.

GRAINS

Many diets will exclude grains due to theory. Some people do well with them, some do not.

There are so many types of grains. Yum! However, some grains are processed and refined to improve their shelf life and texture. They go through a milling process that removes the bran, germ, and all their nutritional value in the process.

Real whole grains are a different story and are suitable for your health. They contain all the nutrients, bran, germ, and endosperm, making it a whole, nutritious food.

We love grains that are sprouted because they tend to be less starchy and have more available nutrients than mature grains do. They also tend to be easier on digestion.

Quinoa is a seed, it is a great grain replacement, because it is higher in protein than a typical grain.

We recommend choosing organic grains and non-GMO, especially wheat and corn.

Healthy whole grains (if tolerated)

- Sprouted grains
- Brown rice (gluten-free)
- Quinoa (gluten-free)
- Oatmeal (gluten-free)
- Organic cornmeal (gluten-free)
- Organic whole wheat
- Bulgar

Unhealthy Grains

- Multigrain
- Grains added to processed foods
- Enriched grains
- Bleached grains
- Refined grains
- White flour

Action:

Now that we have covered organics and the difference between the good and the bad, it's time for another mini kitchen makeover!

Let's pick another five foods that we can switch for a healthier alternative and see how we do.

It's easy to find ourselves attached to certain foods we typically consume, but it's the power of change that empowers us to grow.

If we're ever not satisfied with a new product we have purchased, never hesitate to exchange it for another. Most stores will accommodate. Sometimes we have to try a few before we discover our preferences.

And don't forget! We are worthy, and we are powerful goddesses.

We can repeat the action steps and check-ins as we wish. Once we feel confident, we will be ready to learn all about boosting the immune system for a more profound healing education.

CHAPTER 4

"BOOSTING THE IMMUNE SYSTEM"

"Flushing the Lymphatic System"

Before beginning any healing practice, we must understand the lymphatic system to safely release the body of toxins and get the best results.

The lymphatic system is often overlooked and is almost always found congested in those who suffer from autoimmune dis-ease. The lymphatic system consists of lymphoid organs, lymph nodes, lymph ducts, lymph capillaries, and lymph vessels that make and transport lymph fluid from tissues to the circulatory system. Our lymph is your body's largest drain, it removes cellular wastes, excessive compounds from the digestive tract, and serves as the house of the immune system. Keeping it unclogged will allow our body to release toxins efficiently, so we do not cause havoc on the rest of our systems.

The lymph fluid can contain several substances including, unused proteins, salts and ions, gases and toxic, metabolic wastes, bacteria, fats, dying cells, and immune cells, to name a few.

A congested lymphatic system can cause symptoms such as water retention, bloating, fatigue, joint pain and stiffness, brain fog, cold hands and feet, sinus congestion, earaches, allergies, and acne.

Integrating simple at-home lymphatic flushing techniques in our daily lives can do wonders for our health. Here are a few that we can do regularly for proper natural stimulation.

Rebounding is a technique where we jump on a small trampoline for 15 minutes daily. Any jumping exercise also does this technique.

Skin Brushing is a technique done by using a natural bristle brush by brushing bare skin in a sweeping motion starting at the feet, always brushing towards the heart. We can purchase affordable body brushes online that are specific for the skin.

Other ways include exercise, breath work, lymphatic massage, eating red foods like beets and cranberries, alternating hot and cold showers, and of course, consuming an adequate amount of mineral water for hydration.

Remember, it's never good to detox the body with a congested lymphatic system. We recommend doing research or working with a practitioner when necessary. Yay for health! Now get jumping!

❖

"Juicing Fruits and Vegetables"

Juicing fruits and vegetables is a fun and simple way to boost our immunity by supplying a highly absorbable tonic of vitamins, minerals, and phytonutrients.

Some argue that removing the pulp removes the important fiber, so if we feel our body needs the fiber, then we might want to blend instead. We believe there are benefits to both. We recommend juicing for vegetables like celery, carrots, cucumbers, greens, and blending for foods and fruits such as bananas, blueberries, strawberries, protein powders. Options are endless, and it's always ok to experiment!

There are many juicing trends, including juice fasts and cleanses. We never recommend a fast longer than three days because we have seen people struggle with nutritional deficiencies, that do more harm than good. We support small effective changes.

Juicing can be a fantastic addition to our health and wellness. We can fall in love with juicing vegetables when we don't feel like eating them; however, we do have to keep in mind that juicing vegetables is not an alternative to eating them. Our bodies do need that vegetable fiber. Juicing works great as a pick me up of fresh vitamins, nutrients, and minerals. It's excellent in the mornings; post work out, and perfect for when we're feeling under the weather. If we ever come down with a cold, drinking more than a liter of juice throughout the day can make someone feel much better, much faster.

How do we feel about juicing?

Are we worried that we won't like the taste?

Juicing doesn't have to be an unpleasant experience; with a little guidance, we can create healthy juices that we love to drink. We've put together a juicing guide to guide you and inspire you to enjoy this great addition to your life because the benefits are enormous!

NOT ALL JUICE IS CREATED EQUAL

Pasteurized store-bought juice

Our standard pasteurized juice that we find in a supermarket is made to have a long shelf life. They are typically filled with added sugar, preservatives, and artificial flavor. We want to stay clear of these juices, they hardly have any nutritional value, and they often contain as much sugar as a soda.

Pre-packaged Raw Juice

Pre-packaged raw juices are becoming more and more popular. You can find them at local juiceries, and most health food stores. This is an excellent option for when we're on the go or short of time. Remember to read the labels carefully, choosing raw, organic, and unpasteurized.

Homemade or Freshly Made Juice

This option is by far the most nutritious way to drink the juice. Fresh juice contains the most nutrients. Raw juice bars continue to open up in cities and health food stores. Make sure to ask if the produce is organic for optimum health.

EQUIPMENT FOR HOMEMADE JUICE

There are three types of juicers, centrifugal, masticating, and twin-gear.

Centrifugal is the cheapest and easiest to clean. However, the quick processing, oxidizes the nutrients faster, causing a loss of nutrients in the process.

Masticating juicers extract more juice because they go at a slower speed. We get more nutrition per glass, and the nutrients don't oxidize as quickly. These juices can be stored for up to 24 hours.

Twin–gear juicers are the most expensive of all the juicers, they are the most powerful and can make nut butter and ice cream. They can stay fresh for up to 72 hours.

SOURCE: Kriss Carr's Crazy Sexy Diet; Eat Your Veggies, Ignite Your Spark, And Live Like You Mean It!

JUICING GUIDE

Core Juicing Ingredients:

A handful of kale and or any dark greens
Celery 3-5 stalks
1/2 or 1 Small cucumber
1/2 Lemon with peel

Add ons:

*1 Green apple or pear with core
*1-3 Carrots
^ Handful of Parsley - energy
^ Small amounts of ginger - nausea
^ 2 Fresh beets - immune-boosting
^ 1 or 1/2 Garlic clove - antibacterial

*use these ingredients to sweeten to your taste level and slowly wean off of them due to the high sugar content for boosting immunity.
^ Add these ingredients to change it up or treat symptoms

These are just essential tips; we can get creative and juice just about any vegetables.

- If we have veggies that are about to go bad, let's juice them!
- Have symptoms? Go on the internet and type in "juicing for _____(symptom)."
- Try juicing with only one or two ingredients; sometimes, less is more.
- Get creative and stay inspired. What do you like to juice?
- Reuse the pulp in many recipes.
- Be adventurous.

CITRUS JUICE

Citrus juice is highly beneficial. If we don't own a citrus juicer, we can purchase one at a low cost online. The two main citrus fruits for immunity are lemons and grapefruit; here's why.

Grapefruit

- Highly nutritional, known to combat illness and dis-ease
- High amounts of vitamin C and smaller amounts of A, B complex, E and K
- A large number of minerals, including calcium, folate, phosphorus, and potassium
- Phytonutrients including, limonoids, flavonoids, lycopene, and glucarates, all known to help fight cancer and various diseases

- Has an alkaline reaction helping treat acidity in the digestion
- Contains bioflavonoids known to rid the body of excess estrogen
- Helps reduce excessive amounts of cholesterol from the liver
- Promotes digestion and healthy eliminations
- Reduces fevers
- Alleviates insomnia and fatigue
- Weight loss

Grapefruit in as an acquired taste for some, but the benefits are huge! A favorite immune-boosting drink is fresh grapefruit juice and moringa powder ☺ Google it.

Grapefruit is known to reduce the effects of medication, so we must be wise with our choices.

Lemons

- Flushes out toxins
- Aid digestion and encourage production in bile
- Powerful antibacterial
- Balances the pH level in the body
- Contains potassium, calcium, phosphorus, and magnesium
- Prevents bacterial overgrowth
- Reduces inflammation in joints and knees as it dissolves uric acid
- Helps cure the common cold
- Strengthens liver and enzyme production

• Helps heartburn by balancing calcium and oxygen levels in the liver
  • Prevents wrinkles and acne
  • Nourishes the brain

The best way to consume lemon juice is by juicing several lemons and storing it in a jar or container in the refrigerator. Add small amounts to hot water to drink in the morning like a tea, and also we can use it in salads or in the foods we cook.

"Boosting Immunity"

Pretty much anything plant-based with a bitter or spicy flavor is extra immune-boosting. Unwanted yeast and bacteria in the body thrive off of sweet, starchy, grain foods, and do not succeed in a bitter or spicy environment. Ever had bugs in your kitchen cabinet? What foods did they go after? These foods are similar to the foods that feed the bugs in our guts. Ever use cayenne pepper in a vegetable garden to repel bugs? Again, very similar to how the bugs in our guts work.

Here are some examples of some great immunity-boosting foods; however, there are far more beyond this list.

• Garlic
• Moringa
• Cayenne pepper

- Onions
- Mushrooms
- Dark green vegetables
- Bitter melon
- Lemons
- Cruciferous vegetables
- Oregano
- Ginger
- Elderberry pumpkin seeds
- Pomegranate
- Graviola

Action:

Time for action! What good does any of this education do if we don't act and begin experimenting?

Did we find a juicer yet? Did we make it out to a juicery? If we haven't yet, it's time to make some intentions and follow-through, what we do for our health is entirely up to us.

Have we discovered any new immune-boosting foods that we like or that are perhaps not listed?

"Knowing Acid VS Alkaline"

Cancer and disease cannot survive in an alkaline environment. The best way to understand pH levels in the body is to imagine a swimming pool. If a swimming pool has a low pH level, it means that it is acidic. A low pH would also mean that the pool is more than likely going to be dirty or brown. Now, if the pool is sparkly and clean, it will have a higher pH level and be more alkaline. Try to imagine a body with a low pH. The body would have an overgrowth of unwanted yeasts and bacteria. The best way to keep a clean body is to eat the right amount of alkaline and alkaline forming foods and minimize the acidic ones. We put together a chart so we can get a good idea of which foods are acidic and which ones are alkaline. Immunity boosting foods will always be alkaline and alkaline-forming. We suggest further researching pH balancing, as it is a fantastic way to keep a healthy immune system.

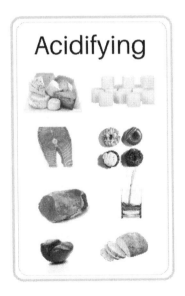

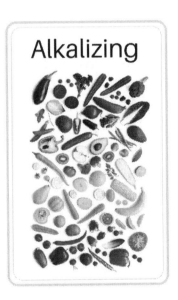

❖

"Understanding Bacteria and Fungi"

If our bodies become too acidic, we'll tend to have an overgrowth of bacteria and oftentimes fungus that goes with it. In addition, if we catch viruses, our bodies will be unable to properly fight the virus, leading to more overgrowth of unwanted microorganisms.

We all have a set of good bacteria and bad bacteria. An abundance of good bacteria is what makes a healthy immune system because they keep the bad ones from multiplying out of control. It's when the bad bacteria start taking over where we begin to have trouble. It's important that we understand and become aware of the different forms of infection. Today most western doctors seem to be over-treating patients with antibiotics in order to continuously kill different forms of bacteria overgrowth in the body. However, they seem to often disregard the possibility of lowering one's overall immune system and the contribution to systemic fungal infections also known as candidiasis.

We can compare antibiotics to pesticides because they eradicate all of the bugs, including the beneficial bugs. Destroying the natural biology in the body causes a number of problems in the body, creating a deficient immune system. It also creates systemic fungal problems in the body that lead to autoimmune diseases, including endometriosis. Learning how to boost our immune system by maintaining a balance of 'good' bacteria can be rather simple. Education is the gateway to living a healthy, joyful life.

"Identifying Candida Overgrowth"

There have been many links between candida and endometriosis. Candida Albicans is microscopic yeast, a normal inhabitant of the human body that can easily become problematic if there becomes an overgrowth. Many health issues affecting women with endometriosis are similar to those caused by candida overgrowth. Candida can reside in our bowels, uterus, bladder, and other organs. Like other funguses, it can plant roots, burrow into linings, and spread throughout the entire body traveling to different organs. Most women have had the well-known and common vaginal yeast infection, but we seem to ignore the yeast infections we can't visually see in our bodies that tend to be just as common.

Unfortunately, when we are being prescribed antibiotics, birth control pills, and pain killers, we become especially susceptible. In addition, a diet high in sugar, and processed foods will contribute to an overgrowth. Sugar and grains are known to feed candida, and actually cause cravings for the foods that feed the yeast. Imagine having a yeast infection in your body that you couldn't see; it then becomes easy to understand how this can be rather painful, causing all sorts of inflammatory responses. Are we starting to see the connection here?

Many women have successfully treated and managed candida overgrowth, have also successfully treated their endometriosis, PMDD, interstitial cystitis, fibromyalgia, and other autoimmune related diseases.

Here are some of the symptoms of candida overgrowth:

* Bloating
* Light red circular rash
* Allergies
* Brain fog
* Inflammation
* Fatigue
* Pelvic pain
* Depression
* Anxiety
* Eczema
* Psoriasis
* Constipation
* IBS ADD/ADHD
* Sugar cravings
* Autoimmune disease

❖

"Controlling Candida"

Candida can be controlled with the Candida Diet, a diet free of foods that feed the organisms by starving them. During this process it is common to actually feel negative side effects from the die off, also known as the Herxheimer's reaction. We recommend researching this before diving into different forms of therapy. In some cases, people can have an overgrowth that may need medical intervention by taking a course of prescribed antifungal. If this is the case, you need to find a well-educated doctor that understands candida. Remember prescription medication is never a cure but rather a tool. We can take an antifungal to rid our body of the yeast but if we don't follow a proper diet and lifestyle, candida can easily just return with a vengeance. We can boost the immune system to keep a healthy properly balanced flora, which keeps candida in check.

It is also important to consider treating any sexual partners where fluids are exchanged. Its possible men can be symptomless and cause continuous infections.

TESTING FOR CANDIDA

The best way to test for candida that we have found so far is a test called, IgG Food Allergy Test w/Candida, found on the website www.greatplainslaboratory.com.

This is a test that can help in more ways than just candida. Food allergens can be a major contributor to poor health.

If we have several symptoms of candida, starting a candida diet will not hurt a thing!

THE CANDIDA DIET

The Candida Diet consists of quite a few restrictions in the first phase of the diet; however, it is only temporary. The diet is free of all sugar, including fruit and sweet vegetable sugar, alcohol, grains, dairy, and processed meats. Also foods like peanuts, and certain mushrooms. They contain mycotoxins that can cause inflammatory responses with candida. If we are serious about combating candida with diet, this is the one diet that could be followed closely for proper results. Never hesitate to get outside help.

Source: Expert Lisa Richards, http:// www.thecandidadiet.com

"Running Off Parasites"

Humans can become easy hosts for unwanted parasites. Yes, we said that right, parasites. Just like our dogs and cats, we can definitely get them too, and surprisingly most people unknowingly have them. If this is new information, we mustn't worry, most parasites are a normal part of our existence and some are actually beneficial.

The second major health issue affecting people around the world today is caused by harmful parasites. Parasites include worms, viruses, and infectious bacteria. Some believe more than half of the human population today has one or more unwanted parasites living in them and neither they nor their physician are aware of it.

Parasites are the secondary cause of food cravings in people with candida. Similar to candida, they leech on the body causing nutritional deficiencies that cause uncontrollable cravings for certain types of foods. These parasites also excrete toxins that can clog up the liver and colon which can easily lead to a weakened immune system and of course the dreaded autoimmune disease.

A strong immunity can naturally rid the body of parasites and keep them at bay, however a weakened body can easily become the perfect host. There are a number of ways one can contract a parasite. They can enter our body through consumption of contaminated food and water, undercooked meat, and contaminated fruits and vegetables. Parasites can also enter our body by traveling through our feet when walking barefoot! We can take supplements or medications that kill the parasites, but we must educate ourselves or work closely with a practitioner to avoid self-intoxication.

Symptoms of a parasitic infection:

* Bloating digestion problems
* Abdominal pain
* IBS

- Autoimmune disease
- Leaky gut
- Nausea
- Fatigue
- Weakness
- Dry skin
- Brittle hair
- Rashes
- Hair loss
- Allergies
- Depression
- Anxiety
- Mood swings
- Brain Fog
- Forgetfulness
- Insomnia
- Teeth grinding
- Weight gain
- Inability to gain weight
- Joint pain
- Cramping
- Numbness of the hands and feet

There are many ways to rid our body of parasites. We highly recommend working with a trained naturopathic doctor for proper diagnoses and treatment.

Source: Amy Myers MD www.amymyersmd.com

❖

"Healing Digestion"

The general talk among health professionals, is that most, if not all, major diseases start in the colon. This is not surprising when we consider that our foods are laced with preservatives, artificial ingredients, hormones, and other chemical additives. Refined, processed, low fiber foods, excessive animal fats, lack of exercise, and an increasing level of stress can all contribute to digestive issues.

Many digestive complaints and symptoms appear even in what seem to be, otherwise healthy people. They frequently go misdiagnosed because the complaints are not "serious". Symptoms such as gas, bloating, diarrhea, constipation, belching, flatulence, food sensitivities, indigestion, malabsorption, irritable bowel syndrome, and the list goes on. They are so common that they are often seen as normal. For some, a sluggish bowel can retain pounds of old toxic fecal matter. This leads to a vicious cycle of autointoxication that taxes our defense systems and eventually leads to more serious disease.

It's important that we take these symptoms into consideration and have education on how to contribute to a healthy digestive system.

❖

"Understanding Enzymes"

"Our digestive system doesn't absorb food, it absorbs nutrients. Food has to be broken down into its nutrient pieces: amino acids (from proteins), fatty acids and cholesterol (from fats), and simple sugars (from carbohydrates), as well as vitamins, minerals, and a variety of other plant and animal compounds. Digestive enzymes, primarily produced in the pancreas and small intestine, break down our food into nutrients so that our bodies can absorb them," says expert Dr. Tim Gerstmar of Aspire Natural Health.

There are many factors that can contribute to low enzyme production including disease, inflammation, toxicity, aging and low stomach acid. Undigested food can contribute to bacterial and fungal overgrowth, inflammation and further digestive issues. It can help us tremendously to up our intake of raw foods that naturally contain enzymes or to add enzymes before meals in order to digest food properly and absorb nutrients more efficiently. We recommend consuming raw foods with every meal, and a full spectrum enzyme before meals. Enzymes work really well for proper digestion.

"Consuming Probiotics"

Now that we know all about the bacteria and fungus that resides in our bodies, it's obvious that we need to supply some of those good bacteria, especially knowing how easy it is to destroy them. Taking a quality probiotic is one way to effectively enhance the body's immune system. Our favorite way to supply probiotics daily is by consuming fermented foods that contain the beneficial bacteria we need. Yogurt contains probiotics; however, it is often contaminated by sugar or lactose that may actually feed the bad organisms, so we must be sure to read the label. Fermented vegetables are filled with probiotics, and are a delicious and effective way to consume probiotics through diet.

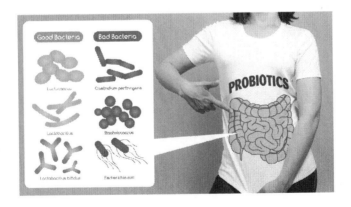

❖

"Avoiding Gluten"

Gluten sensitivity and Celiac disease are on the rise due to many debatable factors. It's important to know whether or not we have a sensitivity because it can very well be contributing to weak immunity. Sensitivities to gluten are widespread in America today; it can give us symptoms of digestive distress, including bloating and painful inflammation if consumed. Gluten can also very well contribute to bacterial and yeast overgrowth in the gastrointestinal tract.

The best way to find out if we have gluten sensitivity is to do an elimination for 2-3 weeks, then reintroduce it back into the diet, and paying attention to how we feel. If interested in learning more about the process of elimination and food allergens, an elimination diet can offer answers.

Gluten is found in foods such as:

- Wheat
- Flour
- Barley
- Malt
- Rye
- Semolina
- Spelt
- Bread
- Pastries

- Crackers
- Cakes
- Cereals
- Beer
- Tortillas
- Soy sauce
- Noodles

Nowadays, companies make a great deal of gluten-free food but don't be fooled by some of these labels just because its gluten-free does not mean its healthy food. We must be thorough when checking labels.

Action:

How's our expert coming along? This is a lot of information and education. What have we discovered about ourselves? Are we taking charge and doing our research? Let's not hesitate to get other opinions, read our information, and experiment.

We can start by writing down three things we are interested in researching and then follow through.

Are we eating more acidic foods, or are we consuming more alkaline foods in our diet? How can we improve?

How do we feel about taking an enzyme and probiotics for better digestion?

Have we tried it? Did it contribute to better digestion?

Do we have symptoms? Ever have any testing done?

Have we tried gluten-free bread yet? Remember to toast it, or it can be crumbly and not satisfying.

Let's create three action steps towards our intentions and make simple changes.
We got this. Life is all about us and self-discoveries.

"Avoiding Constipation"

Constipation is a prevalent symptom, but it is worse for health than one may be aware of. Think about what might happen to stool that sits in our body for more than a couple of days. Of course, it's not something we want to think about, but if there is an issue, it needs to be addressed.

Constipation causes stool to become old, creating an environment for unwanted organisms in the colon. Because the colon is responsible for nutrient absorption, instead of absorbing nutrients, we begin to absorb toxins instead. There are several causes, such as medications or a poor diet that contributes to constipation. We do find that low-fat diets high in processed foods can be a significant contributor.

There are two types of constipation, impacted and residual. Impacted is when someone doesn't eliminate for days or weeks at a time, and the stool is typically hard and dry, difficult to pass. Residual is when there is residual stool being left in the colon, meaning the person is not able to empty their bowels correctly. Both types create a weak immune system and can lead to many health issues.

A diet high in vegetables and plant-based foods is a great way to ease constipation. There are also many natural laxatives and natural procedures that can relieve a temporary issue. However, we highly suggest looking into the culprit before relying on supplements or procedures. Talking to a trained naturopath might be a great place to start.

❖

"Knowing Natural Antibiotics"

As mentioned earlier in this program, antibiotics are very detrimental to an immune system because they act as a human pesticide. They kill all the good and the harmful bacteria, leaving the unhealthy bacteria that are still left to reproduce, creating a stronger future infection that ends up needing more antibiotics. Do we see how this cycle works? As mentioned, this also creates a perfect environment for yeast (candida) to take over, creating a plethora of health issues.

Educating ourselves on immunity and natural antibiotics can play a crucial role in keeping our body free of infection. If we do wind up with an infection, this education can also help us to overcome it naturally. Of course, if it becomes too powerful due to weak immunity and poor nutrition, there may be a need for prescribed antibiotics, and we suggest seeing your doctor.

If a person has to take antibiotics for any reason, we recommend taking a powerful probiotic during and after to restore some of the beneficial bacteria in the gut. Also, avoiding sugar and processed foods is crucial to not end up with another stronger infection. Once we build up our immunity, we will rarely get sick, and when we do, natural antibiotics might do the trick, along with a little immunity support.

Here's a list of natural antibiotics. We recommend seeing a naturopath or doctor for more support, if necessary. Remember, these are just suggestions; there's a lot more to discover and learn about natural medicine, so we are empowering ourselves to get out there and educate ourselves. The earth's natural resources are more powerful than we can imagine, and a whole lot better for our health!

- Garlic
- Honey
- Lemon
- Echinacea
- Pau D'Arco
- Goldenseal
- Oregano oil
- Colloidal Silver

It's important to understand that not all herbal supplements are approved and regulated by the Food and Drug Administration. There is always a concern for mislabeling, compromised quality, and potential adverse side effects. Always look for the highest quality products and do your research to become an informed consumer. Seeking out a trained herbalist is always recommended.

❖

"Detoxing the Body Safely"

When a person has a poor diet, is taking medications, and has weak immunity, there is most likely an overgrowth and accumulation of unwanted bacteria, fungi, and other undesirable substances in the body. When this happens, sometimes we need to undergo a period of detoxification to assist our bodies in creating a cleaner, healthier system.

Detoxification does not take place until the toxicity leaves our body. We can do a whole lot for our immunity by taking herbs, eating better, etc.. However, if we are not eliminating correctly, we can cause what is called autointoxication.

Autointoxication is when we poison ourselves with your own body's toxicity. When organisms die, they emit more toxicity into the system, creating what is also called the 'Die-off' or the 'Herxeimer's Reaction.' There are many ways to make the process of detoxification easier on the body.

We are no replacement for a naturopath or doctor, so we would not be the ones to guide you through detox, however, giving out this information can give us a better understanding of how the body works, when we have the tools to be proactive. We can keep our power alongside a doctor that can assist us.

Check-in:

How are we doing?
How's the education coming along?
Are we making small changes and discovering new ways to boost immunity?
This information is education that can take years to grasp for some fully. If we're facing health challenges, we can remember it's in the inches rather than the huge jumps. When it comes to healing and gaining control over an immune system, we have to be patient and have self-compassion. We are not alone.
Keep strong beautiful! We got this!

CHAPTER 5

"MINDING OUR FOOD"

"Deconstructing Food Cravings"

Cravings... do we dare even mention such a word? What is our outlook on cravings? It seems that the majority of us despise cravings. Cravings are everywhere, just waiting for us to give in. As we give in to these urges, a sudden weakness creeps up on our worth. It's a vicious cycle, and it seems like there is no end. Does this sound like our relationship with cravings?

Let's take a minute to reflect on the human body. Think about how amazing the human body is. It knows when to sleep and when to wake up, maintain the right temperature, and knows how to heal wounds. We genuinely are super humans, with incredible designs.

When it comes to cravings, we must treat them with love and compassion if we want to build a better connection to our bodies. We begin this process of nurturing ourselves with a better understanding of what cravings are telling us. Here is a list of eight possible causes of cravings

1. **Lack of primary food.** Primary foods are areas in our life, such as relationships, connection, spirituality, career, finances, and physical activity. If one of these areas is in the dumps, for example, we are in a negative environment, or we are isolating ourselves and lacking connection, we can crave food or other addictive substances to fill this void.

2. **Dehydration.** When a body is not adequately hydrated, and our body signals thirst, the sensation can also be in the form of mild hunger. It is common for this sensation of dehydration to be ignored, by feeding into hunger rather than thirst. When hunger signals come in, it is recommended to drinking a glass of water before any food consumption or reflect on our water intake for the day and make sure it is appropriate for proper hydration.

3. **Seasonal.** Ever crave foods like squash, baked apples and cinnamon during the fall? Foods like stone fruit and salads during the summer? Believe it or not, our bodies are so smart that they crave foods based on the elements of the seasons on top of supporting our body's seasonal needs. Not

only is seasonal food more flavorful and nutritious, its less on the wallet too. Farmers' markets are great for fresh organic seasonal vegetables.

4. **Lack of nutrients.** If the body is lacking any nutrients, we may crave it. However, oftentimes we go after a non-nutrient dense source to make up for it, creating an imbalance of our body's nutrient needs. For example, inadequate mineral levels lead to salt cravings. We also go after non-nutritional forms of energy like caffeine to give our bodies a false sense of power rather than a nutritious form of energy.

5. **Hormonal.** The fluctuation of hormone levels when women go through menstruation, pregnancy, and menopause cause cravings, alongside with the consumption of added or animal hormones.

6. **Self-sabotage.** A lack of self-esteem and worth can lead to self-sabotage. We crave foods that throw us off, especially when things are going well for us. Creating self-love and compassion with ourselves can help this tremendously.

7. **Blood Sugar Fluctuations.** Eating high amounts of sugar can cause blood sugar spikes and blood sugar lows causing significant fluctuations in moods, cravings, and hunger. A better-balanced diet with adequate raw foods and protein can help regulate blood sugar and ease the chronic hunger sensation.

8. **Overgrowth of yeasts and bacteria in the body.** Many foods feed bacteria and fungi including sugar and processed foods. When there is an overgrowth in the body, these organisms can make us crave such foods for it to thrive in the body happily. This connection can change a person's relationship with food and health if they begin to focus on starving the bacteria and the yeast. They also have more willpower knowing that there is a scientific physical reason they are craving sugar.

Action:

Let's pay attention to the signals our body gives us. Are any of these signals not related to normal hunger?
What is our relationship with our cravings? Do we try to ignore them, or do we feed into them?
In what ways does this lesson help us discover where our cravings might stem from?
What will we do with this education?

"Focusing on Abundance"

As we begin to have a better understanding of cravings, connect more to our food and body, we may go through a period where we feel restricted with food. We start realizing certain foods are no longer serving us, but we love to eat them.

Focusing on abundance rather than lack can help us. It's effortless to focus on what we can't have, but let's take a moment to switch our thoughts on what we can have! Our earth provides an abundance of plant-based foods. Think about it! Do we not live in a world of abundance? Did you know people are more likely these days to know all the brands of jeans and models of cars but are nowhere close to knowing all the different types of fruits and vegetables?

It's time to open our hearts to trying new foods! Have we ever had ice cream made with frozen bananas? What about a Cherimoya? So delicious! We can feel more abundant with food than we did before changing the food we ate and feel far more choices too! Another positive note, choosing is so much easier. Are we starting to feel the abundance and positive changes?

Action:

Let's plan a trip to a local farmers market and choose a few produce items we have never tried before.
What foods might we discover? Who else would love to explore this food with us?

Go online and type in gluten-free, vegan meals, or Paleo if we choose. What recipes pop up for us? Is there anything we would love to make? Let's go for it! Remember to take pictures because I'm sure everyone would like to see it!

Do we have a local health food store? If so, let's take a trip and see what new foods we can discover. Are we afraid we won't like something we purchase? Remember, let's never hesitate to return what we don't like, this helps stores and companies to know what is good and what isn't.

"Minding Our Food"

As we begin to add in the good stuff and become grateful for our food, we also want to consume our food mindfully.

It is very common for the average person to be distracted from the food that nourishes us. Today we have unlimited distractions. Have we ever eaten something and forgotten we ate it? Have we ever driven somewhere and forget how we got there? Maybe it doesn't get this bad, but can we see the correlation here? If we don't give our food the attention it deserves, we often wind up wanting more and more food to satisfy eating.

Mindful eating is so powerful and can be explored on a deep level. It can help us lose weight, eat smaller portions, make better choices, and connect to our food.

We have included an activity that we can do with ourselves or with a partner to enhance our mindfulness when eating.

Even if it's only 10 minutes, let's make time for meals and sit down when eating.

If we turn off the TV, shut down the laptop, and put away the smartphone, we can give eating our full attention.

Action:

Let's reclaim our mealtimes by avoiding eating on the go. Take a moment to see the food. Think about where it came from, what it took to get to the plate. We can look at the color and texture as we smell the aromas. Think about which bite we are going to take first.

As we begin to take our first bite instead of chewing, just let the food sit there for a minute until we start to feel that food and the sensations our body gives us.

When we chew our food, we can pay attention to the texture, flavor, spices, and aromas, chewing our food very well to a puree before swallowing.

Try to focus quietly on the food without any distractions until we have finished our meal.

During our meal and at the end of our meal, let's pay attention to how we feel. Were we satisfied quicker? What did we notice? How did we feel?

"Eating Mindfully"

Mindful eating empowers us with choice by giving us a moment to consciously choose what we put into our body. Consciously choosing when eating food has helped many people become healthier. It contributes to health, weight loss, and helps with food addictions. It teaches us to eat based on internal cues rather than addictive signals, like eating when bored or watching television.

We can control our cravings by being more aware and observant. Paying attention to our food and body allows us to have much more control and connection, leading us to loads of health benefits. How do we think mindful eating can help us?

"Eating Intuitively"

Intuitive eating is different than mindful eating because we are connecting more to our body and our heart to find our truth in what foods we should or shouldn't be eating. It's prevalent for women to have a poor relationship with food when they let their minds, influences, and weak thoughts get in the way of their truth.

We are raised in a society of belief systems when it comes to size standards or diet standards when, ultimately, we need to do what resonates with our best self. What works for someone else might not work for us. Comparing ourselves to others or trying to become exactly like someone we are not, doesn't lead to health or any amount of self-nurturing love.

Principles of eating intuitively include ditching the diet plans, honoring our hunger, making peace with food, discovering satisfaction, respecting our fullness, respecting our body, honoring our feelings without using food, and honoring our health.

Action:

Let's eat the next meal we consume mindfully, but this time pay attention to our food choices. If, for any reason, thoughts come up, observe them.

What is the relationship with our food like? Did any thoughts come up, for example, "I shouldn't be eating this." or, "This food is going to make me look bloated."? Our thoughts are a good indicator of our relationship with the food on our plate.

Let's take a moment to think about the food choices and whether or not our decisions are in alignment with our truth and align with our good health. It's possible that there are times when we have limited options, or we want to experiment. We have to honor ourselves for making the best choice, even if it's not to eat healthily.

We may decide to change what we are choosing to eat; either way, it's all ok, our instinct can tell us whether or not a particular food choice will serve us.

If we're having trouble deciding if a food is going to serve us, an easy way to find our truth is by holding it up to our heart and then asking. Sound kooky? Try it! It works!

These are great ways to get in touch with what foods will serve our health from our highest good. The real work is in the discipline to listen to our bodies.

We may even come up with our authentic ways to intuitively connect to our food. Why not explore?

"Grasping Emotional Eating"

Do we eat when we are stressed? Do we eat when we are full or not truly hungry? Do we eat to soothe a stressful moment? We may want to understand more about what it is to be an emotional eater. Overeating or under-eating based on emotions may not want to be ignored or dismissed when healing from disease. We can obtain more power in our health and life by avoiding acts of emotional eating. Here are some emotional cues, so we can learn how to distinguish emotional hunger from physical hunger. We got this, and we are powerful!

Emotional hunger vs. Physical hunger

• Emotional hunger comes on suddenly instead of gradually. It hits us instantly and feels overwhelming.
• It craves comfort foods, typically fatty, sugary, or salty.
• It often leads to mindless eating and is not satisfying.
• The hunger isn't located in the stomach, and it often leads to regret, guilt, or shame.

"Comprehending the Energetics of Food"

Let's take a moment to reflect on the different energies around us. Energy is a feeling that we get from people and things. It is a feeling attached to what is seen and felt beyond the human eye. We all have different energy at different times. We can even absorb the energy of different people and energy from specific environments. Everything puts off a certain type of energy. This wave can also be called a frequency. Frequency is a vibration that energy puts off, creating the feeling or effect. Can we feel a frequency that the people and things around us put off?

What feels like a low frequency? Do we recognize negative, low energy in a harsh environment? Do we feel bliss by surrounding ourselves with beautiful nature and happy, positive people?

As we reflect on the energy of the things around us, let's begin to take our focus onto the food that we consume. What would contribute to low-frequency food vs. high-frequency food? As ideas may vary from person to person, we must consider this. There can be a direct link to the relationship with our food and the energy of the food we consume.

Factors that may play a role in a food's energy or frequency:

- The health of the food and amount of freshness
- Amount of pesticides and chemicals
- Color of the food
- How the food is presented and looks
- Who prepared it and where it came from
- What it took to get that food to your plate
- Whether or not the food choice is in season

"Food Journaling for Health"

Food journaling is a great way to connect to our bodies. It's up to us how long we decide to do it for, but we recommend doing it for at least three months so we can get a good feel on how our body responds to what we eat. We also recommend food journaling when working with an elimination diet.

Food journaling is rather simple.

As we eat throughout the day, we can pay attention to how we feel 30 mins after eating. During the day or at the end of the day, we can write down everything we ate.

- Liquids
- Grains

* Protein
* Vegetables
* Supplements

We will also want to write down how we feel throughout the day.

* Digestion
* Mood
* Energy
* Cravings

As we journal, we can experiment with food. Each week we can pay attention to how we feel. After a month, we can go back and look for patterns in your moods, digestion, energy, and cravings. Journaling will help us acknowledge what foods work and what foods do not work for us. As we work with mindful and intuitive practices, we can gain strength in our ability to deliver an active food journal. It will also help strengthen our intuition and overall connection to our bodies.

Check-in:

Let's take a moment to check in with ourselves.
How is our relationship with food going?
Are we discovering anything with our food choices?
What have we discovered about ourselves?
Are we feeling more connected to our bodies and the food we are consuming?

In what ways do we feel this has benefited? Is this something we could teach a family member or friend?

What are the five things in our life that we are grateful for?

"Connecting to Our Food"

Most of us live hectic lives, working jobs with long hours, and taking care of families: it's no wonder we easily forget to connect with where our food comes from. Think about how often we get to see how our food grows and meet the farmer who produces it. We get constricted to supermarkets or restaurants where we have no connection to the source. Sometimes we need this convenience, but it is genuinely about the relationship. Once we begin to connect to our food, something inside us shifts. We can follow these action steps for a deeper connection, and we can feel free to share our experience with the world. The world needs it.

Action:

Visit a local organic farm nearby or a Community Supported Agriculture Farm. We can look these up online. They often have visiting hours, or even better, we can volunteer.

We can sign up for affordable organic food delivery. Many local farms have lovely programs that bring fresh vegetables to our doorstep. That way, we can have fresh foods on hand from a source we feel connected to.

Visit our local farmers market! Again, this is a great way to connect to the farmers. Try asking some of them questions about their farm. We can get to know the food purchase and have the freshest vegetables to choose from.

Last, but not least, grow food! Even if it is just a tomato plant or some herbs, growing food is a life-changing way to connect to food.

❖

CHAPTER 6

"AWAKENING THE MIND AND THE SPIRIT"

"Loving Our Mindset"

We might be thinking, how could anyone in pain have a "healthy" mindset? If we feel we are continually not heard, nobody cares, doctors aren't helping, medications aren't working, insurance is not enough, my coworkers don't like me, my boyfriend doesn't love me right, we can be contributing to poor health. Our minds may find us to be anxious about the future or trying to figure out the scary unknown. What did we say wrong? What will we say wrong? Did I or will I fail miserably?   With this mindset, it is impossible to feel proper or safe. A lot of self-doubt, fear, lack of confidence and trust can create a feeble mindset that contributes to an unhealthy body.

Let's use this process to discover where our mind is. Let's be open to addressing our thoughts and learn tools that we can use to shift our mindset, setting us up for limitless potential.

Action:

We can begin by taking moments throughout our day to watch our thoughts. As an author, Eckhart Tolle would say, "watch the thinker."
Let's allow for some self-reflection.
What did we discover about our thoughts? What are our thoughts? Are they fearful, optimistic, worried, negative, or joyful? Let's write in our journal or bring awareness to them.
As we think about these thoughts, where do we feel it in our bodies?
Does this area have anything to do with the location of our pain?
How are our thoughts before going to sleep? Are they repetitive; are they fearful of the future?
What are we discovering about our mindset?

If we give ourselves some time to reflect on our mind and thoughts, we may discover ideas that might not serve us anymore. Together we can take the first step, which is awareness.

"Knowing the Power of Thoughts"

The idea behind the power of our thoughts is based on the concept that, what we continue to focus on, is what our reality can become. For example, if we continuously fear our boyfriend cheating, it can manifest into reality. If we only focus on all the things we don't like, then we may only experience what we don't like. Some of us may even expect things to go wrong before they even happen. This expectation is what we call "preacting" rather than "reacting."

The most significant part of this concept is making a "shift" in our thoughts. Let's do it right now. Take a deep breath. BELIEVE. Through and through, it all comes back to believing. Believing in a positive outcome, believing in the ability to care for our body, believing in others, and, most of all, believing in ourselves. We are so worthy, we are loved, we are light, and we are powerful!

This may not be a shift we can do in an instant, but we have put together tools that can help us shift our mindset and shift our health. Do we believe in ourselves?

❖

"Affirming What We Want"

We are going to start shifting our mindsets by simply adding in good thoughts, using affirmations because we have found them to be very powerful for the mind, body, and soul.

Affirmations are statements located in our minds that claim we are something that we are not. For example, our thoughts may be consciously or unconsciously telling us things like we are not good enough, we're overweight or underweight, we're not beautiful, we're not healthy enough, or not good enough at a particular task. Most of the time, these are deep-rooted lies that we have attached to our thoughts. They stem from somewhere in our past, typically our childhood. These thoughts may also have manifested into a reality. If someone believes in constricting beliefs strongly, they can block anything or anyone from telling them otherwise, and they won't be anything but that belief. Ever tell someone they are beautiful and they instantly say, "No way! I look awful," can't take a compliment? Perhaps this may be us?

Believe it or not, these thought patterns can keep us from achieving optimum health and have been a known link to chronic disease or pain in the body.

We have put together some action steps filled with affirmation examples for better health and wellness. We recommend finding our truth in what affirmations we may need for ourselves and our journey.

Action:

Let's take 5 minutes in the morning or evening or both morning and evening to do affirmations. Some may decide to do them throughout the day. We can say our affirmations out loud; we can also say them while looking into a mirror. We can think of them silently in our meditation or write them in our journal. We suggest experimenting with them and finding our truth with what works for us.
Involving our lives around those who affirm good things rather than those who don't is highly beneficial.

Here are some great healing affirmations for inspiration.

Healing Affirmations:

- I am love.
- I am whole.
- I am healthy.
- I nurture myself.
- I take good care of my body.
- I have compassion for myself.
- I love myself, and I am perfectly healthy.
- Every day I am getting healthier and healthier and feeling better and better.
- Every day is a new day full of health.

❖

"Having Gratitude"

We may not realize it, but something as simple as expressing our gratitude can have such an incredible impact on one's health and wellbeing. Masters have been teaching for centuries that gratitude is a vital component of a happy, balanced, healthy, life. Expressing gratitude to ourselves and others has many health benefits such as less aggression, reduced depression and anxiety, more trust in others, better relationships, and better sleep. Can we see how this might have a profound effect on the physical body?

So, let's begin by taking action and crowding out those negative thoughts with gratitude.

Action:

Once a day, we can create a list of 10-15 things we are grateful for. We can write them, or think them in our thoughts. Feel free to exceed 15 and do as many as we like. We can purchase a journal just for gratitude lists or add it to our existing journal.

As we begin our gratitude practice and start focusing on the things we are thankful for, we can invite ourselves to express to one or two people in our life, and the gratitude we have for them. Pay attention to how we feel, and how the other person feels. What did we discover?

If we are willing, we can experiment with expressing our gratitude to someone who may make us feel a bit uncomfortable. Remember, this is all an experiment, and everything is entirely in our court. We shall only do what resonates with us.

What did we learn from these experiences? We can allow ourselves to receive further education and indeed find our bliss in experimenting with the exercise.

How do we think this exercise can benefit our lives?

"Practicing Meditation"

Our minds can get consumed with thoughts. It's easy to see why we can get so overwhelmed when we're dealing with so much and thinking about so much. Meditation is a simple, convenient, and calm way to calm the busy mind and relax the tension in the body.

There is no one right way to meditate and most people who meditate have their authentic way of doing so. We can start exploring meditation to find what works and resonates most for us.

Let's take this opportunity to pick up a few books on meditation, take a few workshops, watch several YouTube videos, and listen to guided meditations performed by healers. After experimentation and self-education we can discover our true authentic way to meditate.

Here's a recommend meditation practice that we might enjoy.

Through this process, let's find what most resonates with us and find what we desire to carry on into our meditations.

After this simple meditation, we can feel free to explore on our own and keep experimenting with an open mind.

Soon we will be meditating into bliss when our body, mind, and spirit needs it the most.

Action:

In a quiet room or space where we will not be interrupted, let's sit in a straight-up position with the top of our head pointing straight up into the sky with a straight spine. We can sit on a pillow or chair and make our legs comfortable.

Let's bring our focus to our body, observe where we feel tension, and bring awareness to these areas in our body. Observe.

Begin with the top of our crown and start to relax every single body part from top to bottom at a pace that suits us best. Don't forget, the ears, jaw, fingers, and toes.

Let's be still and silent as we bring our focus onto our breath. Is our breathing shallow, or is if full and alive?

As we observe our breath, we can begin breathing deep into our tension areas, starting from the top. As we breathe into these areas, imagine pink light that is healing our body and cells with each breath of air. Let's continue as many cycles of breathing until our body feels open and alive.

Find a comfortable breathing pace and try to imagine or bring awareness to our surroundings. What is here in the room or environment with us? Observe.

Now, let's bring awareness to all of the empty space or the air in our current environment. Try to focus on the opposite of what is tangible. Stay there if we will, for as long as desired.

As we come back to our awareness, we can repeat these words to ourselves or aloud. "I am healthy; I am whole, I am love, and I am light." (These can be your own words, of course.) We can take our time and feel this exercise.

Once we have stepped into this meditation, how do we feel and how is our mind and thoughts at that moment? Do we feel calm, relaxed, or anxious? How long do we think we can rest in this state? Do we believe a meditation like this one will be beneficial to us?
During meditation, we can go over gratitude, affirmations, and higher self-visualization.

❖

"Setting Intentions "

Remember, the term "Thoughts become things." ? When we bring our attention to an intention, we create a thought that lines up with what we want. Rather than focusing on what we don't want, we replace these thoughts with what we do want. With proper focus, we can create powerful intentions.

We intend to nurture our bodies one day at a time and releasing all thoughts that do not serve us. How does that sound to us? Can we feel the power behind these words? What is our sincere intent? Let's be honest with ourselves.

Intentions can be one-word phrases or actions. There are no rules, and of course, finding what works for us is always best. Time to explore!

Action:

Let's take a moment to write in our journal our intentions with each area of our life.
We can start writing our intentions for the day, the month, the year, and maybe five years. We might want to think about this because plans are more powerful than we think.
As we live life, it is empowering and fun to look back at our intention lists to see accomplishments.

We can be free to reflect and set new intentions at our own will and watch our life as it magically unfolds.

"Visualizing Health"

Visualizing health is an ancient technique that is practiced in healthcare. It is a method used for healing, also called guided imagery. If we are not familiar with this technique, it may come across to us as bizarre or wishful thinking, but its effectiveness is validated in dozens of well-designed research studies.

Visualizations can be compelling, much like setting intentions. What we visualize in our minds can give us feelings and reactions internally. These visions create an impression, just the way it does if it were a reality. If we learn how to stay with positive feelings, we can begin to align them with our reality. Are we a skeptic? Why not try it for ourselves?

Action:

Let's sit or lie down in a comfortable position. As we relax, we can bring our awareness to the area in our body that needs healing.

With eyes closed, imagine that area in the body that needs healing, and create a sharp mental picture of what that area looks like.

Now we can vividly imagine that area of the body going through the healing process and what that might look like to us.

Imagine the cells repairing all by themselves, or the toxicity slowly vacating and being whole again, healthy and newly regenerated. If we know more about the healing process, include as many healing details, such as what method the body my need to go through for this healing to take place.

We can get in touch with this feeling of health and imagine our lives in perfect health.

What does perfect health look like to us, and how does it feel? We can allow ourselves to be in this state for as long as needed or desired.

Next, let's try visualizing areas in or life in perfect health, like our relationships, career, and physical fitness. Where can we take this farther, and what can we discover through these exercises?

Source: www.rodalenews.com/visualization-healing

❖

"Understanding Autosuggestion"

As we bring more awareness, as we quiet our minds, we may begin to notice some beliefs and thoughts getting in our way, that we have trouble releasing or letting go. Autosuggestion is something that was suggested to us enough times for the suggestion to be programmed in our minds as real. Sometimes, these suggestions can be tough to let go of. They can become ingrained in our heads and can turn into a block when it comes to our successes. Have we ever assumed we were terrible at something and then found later on that we are not so bad? Do we have thoughts or beliefs that tell us what we can't achieve our dreams? Here's an exercise for us that can help us uncover what has been suggested to us. We can learn how to turn those beliefs into ones that support our deepest desires. We can obtain conceptions that affirm our inner truth.

Action:

Let's begin by taking out our journal. Take a moment to find our center and truth.
Try to reflect on our childhood, school grade experiences, and relationships, if we will.
Write five words we remember people saying to us. Anything that pops up in our head is excellent.
Once we have written our words, let's circle the word that pops up at us.

Let's take a moment to reflect on the word and who may have said this word to us. Where did this word come from, and when was this word suggested to us?

Does this word bring up any emotions or ring any truth to our ears as in something we might believe to be true about ourselves?

Now that we have brought this suggestion to our awareness, we are going to shift this belief from a false opinion and generate a positive recommendation for ourselves.

We can say this aloud if we will or write it in our journal. "In my past it has been suggested that I am _____, this suggestion is false, and it is a lie. I am not _____, I am _____." (affirming the opposite).

We can add this positive suggestion to our daily affirmations, and repeat the exercise when necessary.

"Connecting Our Emotional Pain with Our Physical Pain"

Many of us have emotional pain that goes hand in hand with physical pain. It is easy to see the two as separate, though it is scientifically proven that they are connected.

Emotional trauma can sit heavy in any area of the body. In Eastern medicine, there is a well-known concept that connects physical pain to our body consisting of chakras or centers. Each area of the body holds specific energy, color, expression, or a set of emotions. For example, the sacral chakra is linked to sexual energy, the heart chakra or center would be the love energy, and the throat is communication and so forth. We recommend learning more, as they are a crucial component to health.

Emotions can be painful. Our bodies can feel emotion; do we agree? Where do we feel specific emotions?

Emotional trauma can be deeply rooted in the same way auto-suggestions and belief systems can. Some of us may have gone through trauma at an age where we don't remember. Theories state that it can start as early as in the mother's womb. Trauma can also be a well-remembered trauma that still exists. Most of us have trauma; some of course, may be worse than others; however, we all have it, and we can all overcome it. We are not alone.

What we are discussing is profound stuff. It's emotional stuff that we are carrying around. There is a time where we must let go, shine our light, and move forward.

We wish we could say this is easy 1,2,3, follow these steps, but this isn't typically the case.

To release emotions buried deep, we are going to have to get emotional. We are going to have to feel these emotions and see them and face them as they are.

An accessible route to self-compassion when going through this is to picture ourselves as a baby. We can find our actual innocence and have compassion for our emotions.

Compassion is a window to self-love. Let's embrace the process of release and let go.

During these times of release, as hard as it may be, we highly recommend being alone in a safe environment, unless we have a friend, counselor, or family member that can send us love and light rather than fear or worry. When another person is feeling our emotions for us or magnifying the wrong feeling, this can be an unhealthy energy exchange that can alter our release.

We got this, we are loved, we are light, and we believe in ourselves.

Action:

It's time to dig deep. If we feel comfortable, let's take some time to connect with our family about our childhood. Ask questions about our upbringing and collect any information we may have available.

If we are able, we can explore our mother's pregnancy. We can ask our parents what it was like during our time in the womb. Do we have any siblings? We can ask our siblings about any major episodes or trauma that we may have experienced that we perhaps do not remember. Let's not be surprised about any emotions that come up. When we are too little to understand and feel the feeling, it may be proper to feel it now.

If we want to do this correctly, we highly suggest that we find a compassionate perspective and allow what is to forgive. None of these traumas is our fault, and they have nothing to do with us. Forgiveness, may be one of the hardest things for some people to accept and may take some time to receive, but remember, life happens beyond our control sometimes. And it happens to all of us. Anger and resentment do not lead to health, as love, compassion, and forgiveness for ourselves and others, will.

"Loving Our Job"

Many of us feel stuck in careers or jobs we do not love; we can believe that there is just no way out or nothing better out there for us to do. This attitude may be limiting and could contribute to poor health because we know deep inside that there is always something better. Though, ometimes we may think we don't love our work environment, to find that we can learn to love our jobs by changing your mindset, gratitude, and perspective.

Some of us may love our jobs, but the environment or conditions we work in may not be the best for our health. Our environment can be difficult for someone to bring up or bring awareness to, as we can easily be in denial when we are attached to what we love, or to what gives us a sense of security. Just because we love something or feel secure with something, doesn't always mean that it's serving the highest good. It's up to us what we make of this, and again it is our life. We shall not take advice that does not resonate with us.

If we have a job that we love and that serves our highest good, congratulations, this may be an area that is contributing to health and happiness.

"Creating the Ideal Job"

Action:

Do we know that we have the strength and power to create the job of our dreams? Often it is our belief systems and mindsets that restrict us from doing the jobs that we love to do most.
Let's take some time for reflection or journal writing.
Let's ask ourselves this simple question if we could do anything for a job or career, what would that be?
We can ponder these questions for a while if needed. Nothing has to be answered in any specific timing.
If we are not doing this job or career, what might be in the way?
Let's pay attention to our responses and allow ourselves to observe them.
Are these responses true or false? Are there any negative auto suggestions in the way? Do any anxious thoughts come up?

With the new tools we have, such as intentions, visualizations, affirmations, and gratitude, we can create lists based on any limiting beliefs that come up for us. For example, we may start by expressing the recognition that we have for our job we have now, whether we like it or not. We can create affirmations that affirm the opposite of a limiting belief about ourselves or our situation. We can set an intention to get the job of our dreams or visualize how the position looks and feels. What can we create in our lives?

"Remembering How to Play."

When we think of the word 'play,' we automatically think of children. That's what children do. Play is not just essential for children; it is necessary for adults too: however, we rarely make it a priority.

We can get caught up in our day to day lives, running the hustle and bustles of life. We name it: kids, family, drama, and work. Life can seem like a rat race. It can seem like we can't ever catch up or life decides to throw us curve balls when we least expect it. All that adult stuff takes our adult attention. Most adults will consider play as cutting loose with alcohol or other substances, but how often do we play like we did when we were kids? Sober and adventurous.

It's possible that somewhere between our childhood and adulthood, we have lost our desire for play. Do we remember when playing was not fun anymore? It seems like we don't have any issues with television or computers, though perhaps we enjoy relaxing after all that hard work, and it leaves very little time for active play. It's also possible that we have so many mental distractions with electronics and technology that we can see ourselves and our society missing out on the bliss.

So, let's try to remember this long-lost act. Play is a time where we forget about work and obligations and be alive, fun, and social. There doesn't need to be any point other than enjoying ourselves and what life has to offer. For example, some adult forms of play could be dressing up, playing toss or croquet in the backyard, going on a bike ride or trip to the skating rink, playing a board game at a coffee shop. By allowing ourselves to find the joys in play and releasing what may be holding us back from doing so, we can reap many health benefits and promote wellness and healing. Play can offer stress relief, improve brain function, stimulate the mind, creativity, and improve relationships with others.

Action:

Play.

We are love, we are light, and we are powerful.

❖

"Siding with Nature"

The earth provides an environment for us to thrive; however, it is changing as the world becomes more populated. A majority of us live in cities or suburbs with limited time in true authentic nature. Researchers say that nature has a profound effect on our health and wellness. An unpleasant environment can cause anxiety, high blood pressure, and lower the immune system, and a pleasing environment can do quite the opposite.

When we are in nature, we reduce anger and fear, replacing those feelings with feelings of pleasure. Nature soothes and helps us cope with pain. It also restores our minds, grounds us, and energizes us. We are real nature beings, so much that hospitals and schools have shown that a single plant in a room can have a significant impact on the stress and anxiety of those in the room.

A lack of time in the elements is also known as nature deprivation. Hours spent in front of computer screens or devices have unsurprising links to depression and illness. We can learn to go on hikes, visit lakes, oceans, or waterfalls. We can lay down in a park and watch the trees in the wind.

When is the last time we went out in nature? Is this something that can help us benefit?

Action:

Let's start by taking the time to find a nature spot nearby our work or home that is easy access. We can invite ourselves to visit this spot three times a week if we can make it possible. Let's use this time for a quiet stroll or some silent meditation. Observe nature doing its thing and observe with an open eye, all the details in the plants, the trees, and the sky. It can be as simple as 10 minutes to be with nature, feeling the love it provides.

We can experiment with this exercise to find out what it does for us. How may this benefit our health and wellness? What nature spots do we have further from our home? When is the last time we took an adventurous road trip to a national park?

Finding time for nature can be life changing. We can remember to love ourselves by making time to be in nature. Mother earth provides us with so much healing beauty. We are so blessed to have access to these fantastic healing environments.

CHAPTER 7

"HAVING HEALTHY RELATIONSHIPS"

We are compassionate, nurturing women. It is in our nature to be nurturing to those that love us. However, when compassion only means having compassion for others, we can easily sacrifice ourselves. Let's turn the tables by putting ourselves first, and having the same amount, if not more, compassion, love, and boundaries that we have for others, for ourselves.

If we can learn how to be self-nurturing, we can fill up our own cup and let it spill over onto others. We can feel secure, loved, and care for ourselves with love and understanding, rather than feeling empty and depleted. If we reflect on our mistakes, lessons, life experiences, and hopes with compassion, we might treat ourselves a little differently, and possibly even be treated surprisingly differently by others.

Action:

Here's a simple intro to a meditation that can help guide us to more self-love.

Let's find a quiet space for ourselves without any distractions, including cell phone distractions.
We can sit upright or lie down in a comfortable position.
Close our eyes and imagine we are an angel.

Let's imagine we are an angel above ourselves right now, and we are looking down below. As an angel, we can see our entire life. All of the people in our lives, and who they are, life before and after. This angel that we are can see us in perfect humble light as if we have never changed since we were babies. In the eyes of our angel, we can see our unique innocence.

Now let's look down below upon ourselves and begin thinking deeply about how we could bless ourselves with our own words of nurturing care. What would we say? How would we guide ourselves with motherlike nurturing? Can we imagine ourselves as an angel holding us? What messages would we send to ourselves?

Let's stay here until we feel blessed, loved, and nurtured. This practice can be repeated, as well. We are loved.

Mastering a bond and relationship with ourselves can be made up of many practices. We can encourage ourselves to dig deeper into self-love by reading books, listening to podcasts, and watching YouTube videos at our own pace. This method is just one way and one example.

If we feel discomfort through this process and take responsibility for any feelings that come up, these feelings can provide us with information, by letting us know if we are loving ourselves or abandoning ourselves.

Forms of self-abandonment:

• Staying focused in our head
• Judging ourselves
• Turning to addictions to numb out
• Making someone or something other than ourselves responsible

"Connecting to Our Higher Selves."

There are many points in life where we question ourselves. We can frequently feel lost or disconnected from our truth. We can lose ourselves in relationships and other people's ideas. We can sometimes veer off the path a bit and feel a lack of love from within ourselves. Here's a simple meditation for inspiration. It is just like the prior angel meditation, though this time, we will imagine our higher self.

Action:

Let's Find a quiet space for ourselves without any distraction, including turning off the cell phone.
Sit upright in a comfortable position.
We can begin by closing our eyes and imagine that we are sitting across from ourselves.
Imagine we see ourselves in perfect form. As if this projection has all the answers, it is ideal in all areas of life and is the wisest person we will ever meet; our superpower/superhuman self.
This higher self has access to every memory and positive input.
Take our time to meet this self before us and take time to bond with this higher self.
Begin by acknowledging all the aspects of this self.
Follow through by asking questions, getting advice, and so on. We can meet our higher self that will never leave us stranded. Our higher self will always be there, no matter what.
We can repeat this when we are feeling disconnected from ourselves.

"Believing What is True"

We all grow up with a set of beliefs, whether it's about ourselves or others, we all have them. Our beliefs are set by many sources including, family, media, television, friends, and experiences. However, these beliefs can sometimes hinder us greatly because the idea is not accurate. Let's take our time to dig into our personal beliefs. Often, our beliefs are hidden in our judgments, but not always, our judgments can also be our intuition. No matter what, we want our views to align with our higher self.

It is our job to find the beliefs we have that may be hindering our lives.

Action:

Let's ask ourselves, is it true?
Reach out to a friend or a safe person to talk to about these beliefs. Some beliefs can be so strong they need assistance from another to shift it.
Once we discover what is untrue for ourselves, we can ask a partner to repeat to us what is right.
Reread the segment in chapter 4 on "Auto Suggestion." this section can take us deeper.
Kate Byron is a great mentor for this. She has an abundance of free material online.

"Having Emotional Independence"

After countless moments of feeling like we can't move forward without some intervention, we may wind up driving our emotions deeper. We can use alcohol, substances, and unhealthy relationships to manage emotional pain and suffering, but the consequences often end up uncomfortable and painful. Sometimes it feels like there is no way we can handle our tears on our own or even physical pain without holding someone there with us. We can have deep-rooted feelings that lead us to be needy of the approval from others. Our happiness status can end up being based on what others project on to us. These words might not relate, but this is what we call emotional dependence.

Being emotionally needy and dependent leads us to feel desperate and depressed, affecting our health and wellbeing. If we are always relying on others for our self-worth and emotions, we can be vulnerable to manipulation and heartache. We will go deeper into what independence looks by learning more about interdependence and codependency. If any of this hits home with us, let's try to continue to nurture ourselves in this process. We are not alone; most people in society today struggle with some form of dependency.

Action:

Do we have coping skills when we feel our emotions?
Who do we call when we feel emotional, and how do we feel after the talk?
Is there a healthier person we could contact? Possibly someone not related.

We must have a set of coping skills, and the right people to talk to.

Here's an inspiring list of self coping skills to inspire us to come up with our own or tap into what works for us. Let's act and create a list for ourselves.

- A hot bath
- Essential oils
- Practicing patience with self and the body
- Group therapy
- A mirror pep talk
- Cleaning
- Journal writing
- Playing with a pet
- Time in nature
- Gardening
- Yoga
- Tea
- Games
- Books

"Living Interdependently"

Having interdependence in a relationship is one of the healthiest forms of an intimate relationship. The key to having this type of connection is finding a balance when it comes to each individual's needs. If one person is putting their partner's needs ahead of their own, it can often create imbalance and become a codependent relationship.

Often, when we deny a part of ourselves, we fall into this category by finding a partner to make up for the parts of ourselves we are lacking. For example, an individual could be struggling financially and be attracted to a financially well person, one could find beauty in someone outgoing or funny when they suppress that within themselves, or they could be emotionally dependent. When we bond with this subconscious type of connection, we wind up with resentment. We become enabled to 'not' meet the needs and expressions of ourselves. From here, it's often a downward spiral because our needs are now dependent on this person, including our happiness and our fullness. In return, this person might end up becoming the very one we blame for our unhappiness in the relationship.

If there ever becomes a time where this person can't meet these needs, or they need some time to be alone, it can lead to a feeling of emptiness and loss in the other. It's almost as equivalent to taking a substance away from an abuser. However, if we love and fulfill our own needs, we become more stable and healthily interdependent, giving life to our relationships and ourselves, attracting wellness and wellbeing.

Codependency vs. Interdependence

Many of us may feel confused by the term codependency because, in a healthy relationship, we can feel dependency on friendship, communication, nurturing, appreciation, love, and touch. In a close relationship, we become entangled in meeting these needs of our partners, but of course we are not entitled. However, a codependent relationship will not reap those benefits. They most often relate to others in unhealthy ways with patterns of obsession, self-sacrifice, dysfunctional communication, and control, which is self-destructive and harmful to others.

Here's a list of codependent traits and a list of interdependent traits within relationships. Some of these traits may seem unfamiliar or create a bit of discomfort inside us, but this means that healing is happening as we advance our inner knowledge. Keep on, sister, we got this!

Codependency

- Typically out of balance
- Frequent struggles of power and control
- Anxiousness and resentfulness, feeling guilty or responsible for a partner's feelings and moods
- Control is used to get needs met
- Continuous disagreements and blaming one another for causing problems without taking responsibility
- Feeling trapped in the relationship
- Intimacy may feel threatening

Interdependence

• Power is equally shared, and responsibility is taken for independent feelings, actions, and contributions to the relationship
  • Thoughts and opinions are managed independently
  • Differences are allowed
  • Separateness is honored
  • Intimacy is not feared
  • Independence does not threaten the relationship
  • The relationship gives more freedom
  • There is mutual respect for one each others personal goals.

Source: www.websteruniversity.edu

Action:

Let's take time to go over the areas in our lives where we feel we might be lacking. The life assessment test can be retaken to reassess where one stands.
Make a list of three areas that seem to be the weakest.
Going back to childhood, when in our life have we been enabled or disabled in these areas? Write down under each area what events or circumstances that may have contributed to our weaknesses.
We can ask ourselves what beliefs accumulated about ourselves from the experiences above?
Have we or do we rely on others to fulfill any of these weaknesses or needs?

Let's make a list under each area of 5 action steps we can take in your power to meet our own needs and add strength to our weaknesses.

"Holding on to Our Power."

Have we ever found ourselves in a situation where we feel we have traded our truth for peace and acceptance from others? Do we ever find ourselves relinquishing our power and over-empowering others?

When we do not hold on to ourselves, these encounters and relationships can often bring up feelings of sadness, betrayal, and confusion because we deny a part of who we are. Addiction, unhealthy relationship patterns, financial challenges, health problems, and depression are all signs that we are handing over our power. In this section, we will have the opportunity at our own will, to learn how to protect and own our very own personal power.

One gives away power when:

• In self-doubt
• Trying to make everyone happy
• Over empowering others by looking for approval and validation
• Forgetting one knows what they are doing, and they are good at it.

- Poor boundary setting and honoring takes place
- Allowing self to feel intimidated
- Not honoring and sharing the truth

One keeps personal power when:

- Knowing when and how to say no
- Standing up for self and believing in ourselves no matter what
- Standing on the courage of one's convictions
- Able to ask for needs and wants rather than expecting
- Embracing the fact that one has the right to be respected by others
- Being able to observe behavior without attachment to the outcome
- Spending time with kind considerate people

Source: www.truebalancelifecoaching.com/Shann Vanderleek

Every time we unwillingly give our energy away, we give our power away. When we react, argue, debate, scold, or criticize, we give our power away.

However, if we can realize that we are co-creating every experience, we can reach higher states of wellbeing. We can learn to take responsibility and avoid being in a victim state. This is a core quality of the world's healthiest, most successful people.

Action:

Here is a simple meditation guide or process that can help us overcome giving our power away.

Find a quiet room with no distractions.
We can either lie down or sit for this in a comfortable position.
Take a moment to relax and disperse of distracting thoughts.
Take a moment to connect to ourselves like we did when linking to our higher self in the previous action.
Now, let's ask ourselves, "Which part of us is hesitant to grow? Which part of us knows who we truly are and desires growth?"
Once we can come up with a few answers, let's take ourselves back as young as we can remember.
Let's ask ourselves, what age were we when we consciously gave away our power for the first time? What happened?
Next, instead of visualizing our higher self, let's try to imagine our younger self during this time, and let's invite our younger self to make a different choice. We can do this in any way, shape, or form. Another way is to talk to our younger self with love and compassion, saying words of empowerment during this time.
Let's take time to feel a shift happen within ourselves. This simple technique can have a profound impact on living a more powerful life.

❖

"Holding Ourselves Accountable."

To hold ourselves accountable, we must be honest with others and ourselves. Honesty gets us through our blocks to help us grow. Morality is how we can meet our dreams and align with the right circumstances. When we aren't honest, it emits the frequency of fear. We want to emit a positive frequency to ourselves and others, so we attract health into our lives. We do not want to be stuck, feeling ashamed of our paths, choices, and our desires. We can refuse to have undesired feelings from past instances haunt us by being open and honest.

When we open up to a partner or friend from a place of integrity, it allows room for honesty and openness in others. We can be the ones to plant this seed if it isn't planted already. When we make mistakes, we can say we made a mistake. When we feel we were right, and someone else is wrong, it can create friction. We can still take accountability by saying, "I'm sorry for being a part of this disagreement, can we agree to disagree or meet partway?"

Taking accountability results in loving relationships that can be everlasting.

It can take practice and feel uncomfortable at times, but the results can be astonishing. When we don't take accountability, we often find many things to blame in our outer experience. When we remove blame, we can free up our consciousness to reveal what is causing the blame.

Action :

Find a quiet space without any distractions and take time for reflection.

Use a journal if needed.

Let's begin by being honest with ourselves.
Let's ask ourselves these questions.
What would we like to change about ourselves?
What do you think others want us to change in ourselves?
Do we see any of the things we see in ourselves in others?
Are we compassionate when we see similar weaknesses in others?
Can we treat with compassion, the things inside of us that we sincerely want to change?

This practice can teach us to learn how to be loving with ourselves. Self-compassion is where we need to come from if we want others to be compassionate towards us. We must remove the responsibility we put on others and start applying the responsibility to ourselves.

Here's another set of questions to help us eliminate blame.

When we feel negative feelings in our thoughts, what is typically the reason for the feeling? When we feel irritable, angry, or upset, what is usually the cause?

Write down three things without overthinking, that may be contributing to these thoughts.

Now let's ask ourselves, is it true? Are these things the reason we feel what we feel? Do these things deserve to be blamed? Do we jump around with who and what we blame? What can we change within ourselves, that can help remove undesired blame? How can we move forward with ease and compassion?

"Having Healthy Boundaries"

Have we ever fallen in love with something or someone, and loved it so much that all things other than that love became a nuisance? Do all personal boundaries get loose because what was important no longer stays essential, and our priorities of self-growth are no more because nothing feels better than this feeling of newfound love? It's almost inevitable that we can live this way only for moments at a time before we lose ourselves into oblivion.

Have we ever hit a stressful time in our lives where self-love was pushed aside? Having personal boundaries is honoring our whole being throughout life's ups and downs. When we can't show up for ourselves during our stresses, and we can't show up in our fullness for the things we love, the weights may not get resolved, or the connection may not be lasting. When we show up, and when we feel our best, we can offer real uplifting love to our experience.

Here are some action steps to get in touch with the personal boundaries we currently have, and the barriers we might want to put in place to become a better version of ourselves!

Action:

Let's use a journal so we can make a self-care list.
Let's write down everything we do or want to do for personal self-care.

Let us give some examples:

- A nice morning routine
- 20 minutes of meditation
- A bath
- Yoga
- A healthy dessert
- A weekend at a healing retreat
- A massage
- A meal cooked for us

Please add to this. Circle the ones we would like to do daily.
Underline the ones we can do weekly
And put a star next to monthly/yearly

We can hold ourselves accountable when letting others know. We can inform them and set firm boundaries that we will not sacrifice this precious time. We can let the world know that this allows us to show up healthy. We can build our lives around what matters most.

❖

"Releasing and Preventing Resentment"

Another profound effect of withholding our truth and emotion is resentment. When an outcome doesn't meet someone else's likings or desires, we can easily let it blow over for peace or lack of self-worth, even though we have strong feelings of discontent and pain. We can experience pain by holding it inward, and then find it hard to forgive. When we feel we have been mistreated, judged, or wronged, we tend to have a strong internal reaction. If we want to avoid internalizing this feeling, we must express outwardly what has happened internally by being open with our emotions.

These feelings and emotions can be strong and challenging for one to express because they challenge us to reassess the self-image and expectations we hold for ourselves.

Holding on to such a powerful feeling can quickly and almost always come outwardly with resentment unless released in a healthy, productive, and timely way.

If we choose resentment, it can live inside of us, feeding negative feelings and emotions. The longer it is ignored, the stronger it becomes. Also, it can prevent us from seeing the world from a healthy balanced perspective. Angry people are often living with loads of resentment.

Resentment is a personal feeling. It often affects the person with the bitterness and not the person blamed for creating it. However, it can result in a ticking time bomb for destructive, abusive behavior.

It is common for these habits to stem from childhood. It's often related to growing up in an environment where speaking negative feelings isn't accepted. Also, children often fail to feel they are heard. Another connection to these habits is fear of abandonment. It is not wanting to show one's dislikes or upsets in fear of losing a relationship with the person or having them react in an angry or negative manner and abandon the situation; In other words, feeling unsafe to express negative feelings.

We put together some action tools that support us fully expressing ourselves. Remember that yes, it's good that we focus on the positives in life, but we mustn't deny the negative aspects of experience in the process of doing so. We are both happy and sad, trusting and jealous, calm, and fierce. We are all of these things, and nothing is denied.

Action:

We must learn to express ourselves, so here are some core questions. Let's take our time and open up to our truth.
What kind of life would we be living if we were entirely in our truth?
What negative feelings do we deny having with ourselves or others?
What feelings do we dismiss in others?

What feelings do we have the most substantial judgment?
Are there any feelings that are not ok for us to express?

Here's a simple mantra to better assist expression of feelings:

"Right now, I feel (INSERT EMOTION). I permit myself to feel (INSERT EMOTION) because I have a right to express myself and my emotions."

When we stop trying to control our feelings, life begins to teach us our most important lessons.

Now it's time to get out of our comfort zone and start expressing our feelings; we're not only talking about the negative ones but also the good ones. We would be surprised to know how many people fear expressing good emotions!

When allowed to express feelings, can we express a feeling that we prefer to withhold?
What would be the benefit of expressing these internal feelings with the three main people in our life? What would be the cons?
Are any of these answers untrue?

When expressing a negative feeling toward another, it can be unforeseen when it comes to the reaction of the other person. We can make sure when expressing ourselves that the other person is in the right state of mind, meaning calm and balanced. Our words can have more effects from an energetic, healthy standpoint.

We can try to always talk in the I perspective. Begin by expressing our observation, then our feelings, our needs, and then our requests. This practice stems from the art of Non-violent Communication, a book written by Micah Salaberrios.

Here's an example.

"When I see you are playing video games every night, I feel disconnected because I need a deeper connection. Can we have one or two nights a week game free?"

In our authentic divine power, we can invite ourselves to get out there and start expressing our truth! We got this, and we believe in ourselves.

"Expressing Our True Feelings"

Effects of withdrawal and withholding

We may have all experienced a time where we didn't fully express ourselves and our emotions because we didn't want to be a burden or create any problems. Sometimes it's just more comfortable. Well, the outcome is quite the opposite of easy. When we suppress, stuff, or deny ourselves and our emotions, the consequence is typically just as unfortunate as the consequence of an anger outburst. Communication is a tool we have to connect us to others as well as ourselves. If we don't use the tools correctly, we wind up disconnected from ourselves and others.

We as individuals can choose to communicate in a way that restores our sense of safety and love connection to one another, or we can select defensive strategies that increase the distance and sense of loneliness or anxiety from a feeling of disconnect.

When we choose to disconnect, we often find ourselves with a partner that intensely reaches for a closer connection. A disconnected withholding relationship can lead to a plethora of problems leading to acts of anger, fear, and even rage. It is never a good idea to leave the painful emotions to the subconscious. It is much easier to live our lives consciously aware of our feelings, to be willing to feel our souls, and to be ready to put our feelings into words when possible.

Our emotions and feelings are our teachers, our guides, and our important messages to us from our bodies. They let us know where we are in terms of where we want to be. If we can listen, we can begin to fully understand, accept, and connect lovingly with ourselves and others. Expressing emotions allows us to build trust and safety in relationships.

It's essential to know the reasons why we suppress emotions. Somewhere along our path, typically stemming from childhood, there is often a pattern that begins due to the lack of feeling safe to express feelings. As a child, it may have worked for us to become defensive and protective, creating a habit. However, in an adult relationship, this technique often keeps partners in survival mode, building distance between them.

Emotions can be put into two categories, being either fear or love based. Fear emotions and related emotions of shame and guilt are frequently the feelings that put distance keep us apart. However, at the same time, the concerns we bring awareness to can give us vital information on what each partner yearns for. Our fears drive us to our core emotional needs, being as real as our needs for water, food, and oxygen.

Action:

We can choose someone in our life that we have a close relationship with or someone we desire more intimacy with. Someone we know well and have spent some time with like a family member, spouse, boyfriend, close friend.
Let's pick five feelings that we have about this person that come from love and write them in a journal or on paper.
Next, pick five feelings we feel from or about this person that may be of fear. Let's be honest with ourselves.
What feelings in both categories do we feel like we can't express easily, and which emotions do you think we can communicate. What feelings might be more challenging or feel unsafe to express?
Can we explain to ourselves why these feelings may be easy or difficult for us? Are any of these beliefs correct?
What benefits do we think the relationship will receive if we willingly speak up about any of these feelings we might be withholding?

How might we bring a stronger connection to our relationships?

"Accepting What Is"

When we can accept the way things are and learn to have gratitude for what is, we can release a lot of much-needed suffering. Being that we are on a healing journey, it is extraordinary to think that we are going to look back on this moment with more wisdom and grace.

If we compare ourselves to others that we feel are more advanced, we can feel negative feelings of what seems like an unreachable desire. We might quickly get in our way, and wind up removing the compassionate self that understands that it is our journey. We can learn that the prize is not something that is handed to us, but it exists in the process of being wowed by our revelations.

We hope we can find peace and be humbled by our experiences no matter where we are.

Action:

Let's write a love letter!
We are going to write a letter to ourselves as if it is ten years in our successful future, and we are writing to ourselves currently.

To make this even more powerful, we can have a partner read it back to us.

This letter is intended for us to see our current circumstances with compassion and light. To be humbled by where we are at today and what is, because deep inside, we all know we are going to fly, and this moment won't last forever.

"Coupling and Uncoupling Consciously"

Ending a chapter in our lives can feel devastating, especially when it involves leaving a partner we built our lives around. Change can be scary, but we know deep inside that the changes we create for ourselves are the very ones we need to grow. Either way, breakups are never easy, but do they have to end so abruptly? Do they have to involve so much of a loss? Does our greatest fear need to become a reality? Maybe not.

When we become angry or feel at a loss, we can believe that the quickest relief to removing these painful feelings of hopelessness is to lose it all and start over. These feelings are more likely to happen when we feel sensations of fight or flight. We want to end it all right then and there because we feel hopeless in that moment.

We can begin by allowing ourselves to be ok with these thoughts. We can panic less by learning to cope with unwanted emotions. We can learn to make drastic changes outside of this feeling of fight or flight by waiting for it to pass. Our thoughts can be irregular, irrational, and they might not always align with our higher selves when we are upset. Also, these feelings of fight or flight might stem from the past, so it's essential to be in a healthy state when making big decisions.

A relationship ends when we are unable to have the most needed conversations. We can learn how to open up and speak our truth when we are calm and cope with self-love when we are not. We can practice this with a partner by opening up time for truthful conversations when we feel our best. Learning how to offer each other space for self-love and providing love and support when things feel off, rather than engaging in life-changing conversations.

We mustn't fear loss, because even if we decide to go separate paths, the relationship can evolve apart, or it can be an everlasting friendship. We all make mistakes for many reasons; if we can be 100% honest with our partner, we can access what we need to gain for growth, whether it is apart or together. If it is alone, we must know that our truth will align us with what we desire most by making positive changes. We can love one another through change. Love can stay unconditional.

Action:

How can we be more honest with ourselves when it comes to expressing our most authentic desires?

We can love our journal by writing down five of our biggest love relationship desires and friendship relationship desires, even if they are already fulfilled. We can open up this awareness.

Now we can take the time to think about expressing these desires to our closest ones. Do any feelings come up?

If we feel a flutter, anxiousness, or discomfort, we can learn to dive deep into what might be hindering us from our loving expression.

We can begin by taking time with a loved one when we feel great, perhaps lunch or tea. We can use that time to express gratitude and possibly expressing any needs or desires within the relationship.

By taking the time, we can avoid withholding feelings and desires that may lead to feelings of hopelessness.

"Honoring Our Temple"

If we had our own temple, how would it look? Who may we invite in? How would we protect our temple? How would we care for it? How would we honor or adorn our temple?

These are all great questions if we can see that our body is our very own temple.

If we want to love this temple of ours, indeed, we must honor it. We have to care for its appearance. Be aware of who we want to attract, know to keep it healthy, keep the bad folks away, and keep it safe!

It's wild that we can often find ourselves having to remember how to care for the very thing that gives us life in this physical world. Sadly, our bodies did not come with a manual; however, if we can answer these questions, we may be able to tap into genuine nurturing of ourselves. We can learn how to truly represent from a self-nurtured place, offering ourselves an upgrade, and more safety from harm.

Action:

Let's meditate on this reading for a moment.
We can imagine our temple perfect and whole.
Let's take a moment to think of all of our acquaintances, friends, exes, lovers.
Who do we let in close to our temple? Who do we keep at a distance?
In what ways can we adjourn our temple?
Is it wearing enriching face oil, elaborating with eco makeup, being bold and flashy with our appearance, or blending in with the earth?
How can we honor our temple to align with our values?
What changes can we make?

CHAPTER 8

"NURTURING OUR WOMB"

"Learning About Hormones"

Our hormones are chemicals made within our bodies created to support and protect life. They are responsible for procreation, attraction, fight, flight, and growth. They regulate our cycles, our heart rate, sexual function, mood, and temperature. It's no wonder we can feel an incredible amount of sensations when our hormones are over or under-active.

Hormone imbalances can be genetic, food-related, caused by birth control use, or from environmental factors.

We hope to imply the importance of regulating hormones by taking hormone tests, learning hormone balancing knowledge, and having awareness. When our hormones are off, or they fluctuate to uncomfortable measures, it can bring in a plethora of symptoms.

Symptoms include:

- Overly or under-active libido
- Fatigue or restlessness
- Anxiety
- Depression
- Moodiness
- Irritability
- Irrationality
- Hot flashes
- Heart palpitations
- Weight gain or weight loss
- Headaches
- Panic attacks
- Victimhood mentality
- Vitamin deficiencies
- PMS
- PMDD
- Autoimmune dis-ease

Unbalanced hormones can affect our lives and be challenging to pinpoint and understand. We can learn and grow a lot by getting our hormones tested and by working with a practitioner for a better understanding of our bodies and symptoms.

As a woman, we naturally fluctuate. Our hormones are one of the first things to be affected when our body undergoes any stress. We deserve to feel good and understand our bodies.

Our menstrual cycle has phases including menstruation, the follicular phase, the proliferative phase, ovulation, the luteal phase, and the secretory phase.

During menstruation, levels of estrogen and progesterone are low. The Follicular and proliferative phase is before ovulation. The lining starts to build, in order to shed again, and estrogen slowly rises. Ovulation is the release of the egg. Estrogen peaks right before ovulation and then decreases shortly after. Progesterone peaks in the next phase, which is the luteal phase. This is when the body prepares itself for a possible pregnancy. In the secretory phase, the body will produce a chemical to support fertility, or it will prepare to shed the uterine lining if pregnancy does not occur.

It's familiar and can be natural for women to feel the fluctuations in hormones. During our ovulation and luteal phase, we can feel more sensitive, need more time to ourselves, and desire more self-nurturing and peace. We do not want to withhold feelings or lack personal boundaries during any phase because feelings can build up and backfire during this sensitive time where we can't hold anything back. Can we see how it is possible that withholding feelings can contribute to irregular cycles, including PMS. Sometimes it's challenging to speak up because we don't want to upset anyone, but we can love ourselves better when doing most of our movements of energy in the phases we feel our best.

Action:

Have we ever had our hormones tested? Life Extension is a company that offers affordable lab testing for just about anything. We can see our results within a week and talk to a specialist about the results. Another option is to contact our doctor or naturopath. A preferred doctor or naturopath can give us valuable information. Testing is a great way to become deeply connected to our bodies.

Here are a few questions to ignite a happier flow!
Is there anything that's bothering us?
When is a great time to discuss it with someone?
What phase are we in?
Have we tried a period tracker phone application?

"Dominating Estrogen Dominance"

Estrogen helps our bodies initiate sexual development, while progesterone helps us regulate our menstrual cycle.

Estrogen can become dominant from environmental stresses on the body that can be caused by the intake of synthetic hormones, including birth control, the consumption of foods high in phytoestrogens, or synthetic hormones. It can also be genetic. How was the reproductive health of our mother or grandmothers?

Estrogen dominance has become a common factor in reproductive issues.

We recommend eating a balanced diet, avoiding foods high in phytoestrogens, or synthetic hormones found in dairy and meat. A menu full of cruciferous vegetables, legumes, seafood, and complex carbs, while avoiding alcohol, caffeine, soy, and refined sugar.

For stubborn dominance, supplements and vitamins worth researching are:

• Vitamin D
• Vitex
• DIM
• Calcium D-Glucarate

Action:

It's time to adjust our diet if needed.
Let's be kind to ourselves and swap three foods we love to consume that might contribute to estrogen dominance and replace them with delicious foods that help balance our hormones.

Hormone balancing foods:

- Salmon
- Hemp
- Cruciferous vegetables
- Legumes
- Nuts
- Avocados
- Leafy greens

Estrogenic foods:

- Soy
- Processed foods
- Synthetic hormones in meat and dairy
- Caffeine
- Refined sugar
- Alcohol

"Caring For our Reproductive Organs"

Our sacred womb, our ovaries, our uterus, our cervix, our vulva desire to be cared for in ways we may or may know. The door to the deepest part of ourselves wants to stay sacred and nurtured for optimum health, so we must know more.

We know to avoid certain soaps, but what about the things that we don't always talk about or truly grasp? Is there more to caring for this part of ourselves?

Here are some factors that can affect our reproductive organs that our mother may not have known to teach us.

Bacteria can create a problem when cleanliness is an issue, but typically bacteria is a common problem caused by sexual intercourse. When we exchange bodily fluids, we have to be clean, or all sorts of things can happen. If bacteria affect the vagina, it can travel to the cervix, cause cervicitis and affect our menstrual flow resulting in retrograde menstruation, which is a leading disruption behind endometriosis. Sometimes we won't have symptoms with cervicitis, and an infection along with inflammation can fester, leading to more significant issues. We have to be wise and care for our womb in the best way we can. If we ever notice a change in odor that doesn't go away, typically after intercourse, we must never ignore this. We recommend seeing a doctor or researching the use of boric acid suppositories if this happens. We will also probably want to confront this issue with our partner and only have protected sex if this is a constant issue or until the issue is resolved. Men can unknowingly carry bacteria in their sperm that create disease and infertility in both partners.

Yeast infections can happen from consuming too many sugars, or carbohydrates. They can also occur when there is too much moisture from wet clothing, gym clothes, or bathing suit. But, what we don't always address is that yeast infections, also known as candidiasis, can come from intercourse with male ejaculation. Men that consume large amounts of sugars or alcohol can have an overgrowth of yeast in their bodies, including in their sperm. So, if we notice infections happening with intercourse, this must be addressed.

Yeast is no joke and should be treated in both partners when necessary, as it can also inflame the cervix resulting in dis-ease if untreated. If this is a repeated problem, it is essential to confront our partners, contact a doctor or naturopath, alongside with researching the occasional use of boric acid suppositories.

We want to keep a healthy biome in our inner workings. Unwanted factors can all create an improper pH balance that could be hard to maintain without proper care. We must honor these organs and honor our temple.

Action:

We can research boric acid suppositories and have a plan in place when things feel off, so our organs are never left untreated.

❖

"Living Within Our Natural Cycle."

Humans are cyclic, and so is the entire universe. Every moon, we change and evolve. Women are highly in tune with cycles as they have a direct reproductive cycle every month. Men can connect to the cycles through Mother Earth and are also known to have a cycle as well.

Some theories say we can sync with the moon by ovulating with the new moon and menstruating with the full moon or by ovulating with the full moon and menstruating with the new moon. The lunar cycle is 29.5 days, and the average menstrual cycle length is 29 days. Insects and animals tend to reproduce on full moons. What does this say about our cycles?

Our environment can change so drastically through the seasons; we can change drastically too. Just like the trees, we change as we move through the changes in temperature. We can embrace when the veils become thin during the transition. We can take our time to remember the past seasons; we can embrace a new time; we can shed what no longer serves us and open up to the new.

In times of emotional change, remember all it is, is energy in motion. Sometimes we can try to attach these emotions to our outer experience. However, we can rest assured when we realize that it's merely change happening on a universal level, and it is a special time of remembrance. Even if it feels sad, it can all be for good reasons.

Action:

Journal writing questions for research and thought:

Do we track our cycle?
Is our cycle close to 29 days?
Does our cycle correlate at all with the moon cycles?
What changes for us when the seasons change?
Do we feel the new moon or the full moon?
If emotions are energy in motion, how can we better perceive our feelings?
Do we notice the cycles in nature?

Find a nature walk to go on at least twice a week. Take note each time we notice the natural changes that take place. We can be sure to go to every full moon and new moon, if possible. We might be amazed!

"Being Curious About the Feminine and the Masculine"

The sweet nurturing, divine, graceful, elegant, feminine woman and the raw, charged, dominant, protective, humble, handsome, robust, masculine man; how is it feasible for these two roles, whether they are scientific or societal differences, to come together in harmony? Can we be curious about these relationships and learn the differences?

A man offers his life energy to the feminine during sexual intercourse when he fertilizes her eggs, for the reproduction of human life! It's quite a profound ability we have to create when we connect! When a woman goes through her changes to support life in her womb, or she is naturally sensitive because her body is doing the work to support another life. The masculine fulfills his role when he can protect and keep his impregnated woman safe. These roles are a more natural way of looking at our innate functions as humans. If pregnancy does not happen, it seems reasonable to believe the fulfilling roles between the masculine and feminine can be practiced regardless, giving the relationship the ability to thrive when they are acknowledged.

The man can learn how to offer safety to the woman during her sensitive phase by understanding her sensitivity. We can let the man know that this phase is not a time for debate or time to challenge the sensitivity but rather a time to listen, nurture, and offer safe, loving words; a time to avoid unnecessary stressful conversations and business matters, unless they are approached sensitively and compassionately.

If we are not upfront about our changes and fluctuations, sensitivity can often be confusing to men. The man can withdraw from sensitive energy and bring on feelings of insecurity when it comes to the relationship. Women do not want to go through that. We have to make sure the men can read past the irritability and bitch face that comes from rushes of hormones and sensitivity and not take it personally. We want them to continue to feel loved, secure, and learn how to understand us. Men can learn to continue to offer love, touch, and safety during this time. They can feel that they are fulfilling an innate role, which might bring on a more solid relationship.

"Having Healthy Intercourse"

Healthy intercourse lies in cleanliness, protection, and not having multiple partners. However, some people might not see how a lack of connection and fear of intimacy could contribute to unhealthy sex as well.

Our lives are so busy, sex gets repetitive or none-existent. We might only feel safe with unavailable partners, or we might only feel safe with multiple partners. When these things are not addressed in partnerships, sex can become painful, especially for a woman.

A disconnect can often leave small talk and foreplay at bay. When we do connect, it can be rough and to the point. This type of sex can feel good, but there is a chance that we might have some unhealthy sexual habits that may or may not work for us.

We want to honor our temple. When we have mindless rough sex, we can damage our organs that we need to care for properly so we can have a happy, healthy reproductive cycle. We can let our partners know how sacred our bodies are, especially our womb. If we open up about these needs, we can teach the masculine energy to connect to the divine feminine. We can let them know precisely how to communicate with us. Take care and allow time for natural lubrication by having more small talk between connection and foreplay. The cervix can stay healthier with the right lubricant. The cervix can also feel good with pressure, but we must remember not to be too rough and hurt this area because it causes inflammation that can affect our flow.

A lot of information! We wouldn't be here if we weren't ready for it! And remember this is all take it or leave it, not all of it is science-based information, that is why we do our own research and decide what we will.

Action:

Let's invite ourselves to add one of these healthy acts each time we connect with a partner.

- Massage each other
- Foreplay
- Small talk
- Eye contact
- Kissing
- A new face to face position

If any of these new acts become uncomfortable for either person, it shall be approached gently, lightly and slowly. Some people can take more time than others to feel a deeper connection. We shall be patient and continue to offer safety. Deep intimacy can feel unsafe for some, but we can overcome it with compassion and grace. Some people have been avoiding deep intimacy for many years, or perhaps they have never experienced it.

"Healing Sexual Trauma"

Often, we may not know that we are being affected by past sexual trauma until it shows up in our sexual relationships.

Sexual trauma can come from childhood and adulthood, and typically comes from non-consensual acts. When this happens, it can show up as anxiety when sex is initiated or acted similarly as the non-consensual act. It can lead us to feel safer with unavailable partners or eventually completely shut off to available partners to avoid this anxiety and discomfort that comes from a similar act or approach. This anxiety can happen even when the new connection is consensual and safe.

When we open up about our experiences to our partners, we can also open up about what offers us safety during individual acts. Sometimes, if we know that our partners are aware of what happened, or we bring awareness to where our reaction stems from, it can make all the difference for us to feel safer. If we need to have boundaries and approach something slower, our needs shall be honored. If a person oversteps our limitations, we might want to move away from or heal the relationship we have with this person to avoid being triggered and creating more trauma. With the right partner, we can learn to feel safe again.

Action:

Love ourselves.

Join us! This book is available as an eCourse and membership at www.HealthByHer.com. We offer support groups, extra education, media, recipes, Amazon health product recommendations, articles and more!

Made in the USA
Middletown, DE
01 June 2020

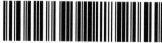